FOUR Ts

TO A BETTER YOU

A BLUEPRINT FOR IDENTIFYING AND ADDRESSING
THE FOUR CAUSES OF SICKNESS

READE L. HUBERT, DC

Dedication

To the people who got in my way,
and to those who showed me the way.

CONTENTS

PREFACE

BEFORE YOU DIVE IN, I would like to give a nod to the many men and women who contributed to the incredible field of chiropractic before me. I couldn't have written this book without the many pioneers in the field, and I salute them for their pivotal contributions.

As the saying goes: *I stand on the shoulders of giants.*

While this book is a distillation of the knowledge I have gained over the past twenty-five years, I took a few, well-known concepts in chiropractic—two in particular—and expanded on them.

This book details how every ailment can be traced back to the Four Ts, but the first three Ts—thoughts, toxins, and trauma—are nothing groundbreaking. In fact, they are staples in my profession. Talk to any chiropractor and they will immediately recognize these terms and understand their significance.

D.D. Palmer, the founder of chiropractic, first wrote about thoughts, toxins, and trauma in his book, *The Chiropractor's Adjuster*, released in 1910—although he didn't refer to them as the Three Ts. Later, in 1921, his son, B.J. Palmer—also a chiropractor—re-released his father's book (with some editing) and called it, *The Chiropractic Adjuster*. I've taken what was previously written about thoughts, toxins, and trauma and have presented them in a way that makes sense to you *today*.

While the first three Ts are not new, I am the first (to my knowledge) to add the fourth T: traits—i.e. genes. With the rather recent emergence of science regarding genetics, our genes and how they are expressed cannot be ignored when assessing our health through a holistic lens. The fourth T was the missing link, and now, along with the prior three Ts, I present an all-encompassing approach to find the root of our sicknesses.

Another early concept within chiropractic is the concept of time. We have a saying, found in principle number six: *Every process takes time*. In the pages that follow, you will see that I expand on this concept and make it timeless to the health issues we are currently dealing with.

My goal was to broaden and enhance old teachings by making them relevant to today's standards—including incorporating recent scientific studies and advancements. The result is the book you hold in your hands.

INTRODUCTION

NOBODY HAS PROBABLY TOLD YOU, but you've been approaching your health all wrong.

It's not your fault, though. Our society's contemporary approach to health has complicated it for you. Even the World Health Organization (WHO), the eminent global health champion, offers a useless definition: "Health is a state of complete physical, mental, and social well-being and not merely the absence of disease or infirmity."

A "state of complete well-being"? Well, it's no wonder why the average person without a medical background doesn't understand what good health is and how to get there. The WHO's phrase of a "state of complete well-being" implies perfection—which right out of the gate is problematic because it is impossible. If you can't scientifically define well-being, how can you begin to address it?

And don't get me started on Dr. Google.

Although the internet has its perks, using it when it comes to anything health-related usually ends in disaster. At best, people searching for answers on how to improve their condition often end up overwhelmed, confused, and frustrated. At worst, they take what they read online as gospel and end up worsening their situation.

Most professions within the healthcare community are working in a broken, expensive, and tired model. We are more concerned about effects than causes. Well-educated, well-intentioned, but wrong.

To start approaching health properly, we need a new, simpler, individualistic, and achievable definition:

> *Health is feeling the best you can, where you're at, without the expectation of perfection.*

In other words, health is about *a better you.*

A better you will look different to everyone. A twenty-year-old, for example, may want to run a marathon whereas an eighty-year-old may just want to get out of a chair with ease and walk to the refrigerator without losing his breath. If both of them feel good doing what they want to do, given where they are in life, then they have health.

A better you is within your reach, too, regardless of your age, season of life, or diagnosis.

A menopausal woman who walks into my practice for help with fluctuating hormones and hot flashes, for example, can't expect to feel like she's thirty again, but she also doesn't have to suffer. Perhaps a personalized and specific care plan can help her; she can make decisions that lead to feeling better.

Conversely, a terminal cancer patient given weeks to live can still feel joyful about making it to another day.

Health is not about perfection. The WHO misses the mark with their definition, and in fact, may even do us a great disservice.

Health is simply about *a better you*—and getting there is easier than you might think.

YOU ARE DESIGNED TO BE WELL

We need to stop looking at health as something everlasting—because it's not. You are made up of borrowed materials—literally from the dust of the stars—and you will have to give them back to the planet for future generations to use.

The physical universe is constantly trying to break you down—whether that's through harsh weather, malnutrition, pollution, workplace stress, or various viruses and bacteria. I call this process *universal composting*.

But here's what is often woefully overlooked: your body is an amazing instrument of creation capable of, and specifically designed to, help you overcome whatever comes your way.

This may come as a surprise to you, but you are *designed to be well*, not sick.

Your body is a closed system of animated matter that has the incredible power to take care of itself. You are designed to go until you cannot go anymore and your cells switch off, at which point everything that makes up who you are will be recycled. Your flesh, bones, cells, and minerals will go back to the ground, back into the water, or back in the air. It happens to everybody—past, present, and future. We're breathing some of the same air molecules Gandhi, Christ, Cleopatra, and all your genetic ancestors breathed.

When our bodies can't keep up with the external pressures, we get out of balance. Disease then sets in because we don't give our body what it needs to thrive. Yes, the universe is constantly trying to break us down, but by treating the body well and reducing stressors, we can protect ourselves and set up our bodies to do the incredible things they're specifically designed to do.

We have to stop looking at our bodies as the problem, and start believing our bodies are the solution—given that we're creating an environment our bodies need to succeed.

Every decision we make in our lives causes either a positive cellular change—where we resist universal composting—or a negative cellular change—where we usher in illness. Once we're aware of this, we can make decisions and do things that keep our bodies functioning the way we want them to so we may enjoy fuller, happier lives the way we were intended.

Maybe you don't feel well because you've been struggling with imbalance within your own body. Perhaps you're caring for loved ones—your significant other, your children, or your aging parents—and you want to do everything you can to alleviate symptoms and help them feel better, but you don't know how.

Starting now, you can put everything you think you know aside and begin paying attention to what really counts. I'm here to teach you that health isn't *that* complicated, because every disease or disorder can be traced back to four root categories of cause—thoughts, toxins, trauma, and traits.

You can slow down universal composting—and in some cases, completely stop it—by focusing and working on the Four Ts. Every time you improve these areas, you're creating positive change at the cellular level, and you'll end up being *a better you.*

True success is positive cellular change. When your body adapts positively, you win.

Whether you're dealing with high blood pressure, diabetes, genetic disorders, long-term COVID-19 effects, or any other condition, understanding the Four Ts is the key to *a better you*.

INSIDE THESE PAGES

When it comes to the volumes of medical and health information out there these days, I like to picture a funnel. That information tries to enter at the top of the funnel, but it's too much. This then leaves you confused and outraged, not knowing where to even begin.

This book will show you how to stop engaging with your health at the top of the information funnel, where there's too much to process, and instead simplifies what you need to know by focusing on the bottom of the funnel. Here is where the profusion of mind-boggling information gets narrowed down into four easy-to-grasp categories—thoughts, toxins, trauma, and traits. By focusing on the bottom of the funnel instead of the top, you will feel empowered, inspired, and relieved—and you'll be well on your way to *a better you*.

In the pages that follow, you'll learn about each of the Four Ts, along with how all four of them interact with each other. Health is not linear, and every T layers on top of another. But for the purpose of introducing each category, I've dedicated one chapter to each T.

The first **T** is *thoughts*: The mental processes that give rise to positive (or negative) cellular change. The cellular machinery in your brain is responsible for making a thought happen, but you don't have full control over this, which can affect your health. You need proper, positive mental stress to adapt and be better, which we'll explore in Chapter 1.

The second **T** is *toxins*: Matter we put into our bodies (via food, water, air) that the body is unable to deal with causes a negative cellular change. Humans have polluted nature, and that pollution brings toxins into our bodies, causing disease. It's imperative to find ways to overcome the microplastics we consume, the forever chemicals in our drinking water, the toxins we breathe in from polluted air, and other pollutants we absorb. We will discuss these, and more, in Chapter 2.

The third **T** is *trauma*: A negative cellular change arising from a lack of physical matter in the body—although in certain circumstances, this can also produce a positive cellular change, which we will explore in Chapter 3. The body can take quite a beating. But your body has an amazing ability to adapt and overcome.

And finally, the fourth **T** is *traits*: Your downloaded hard drive of genes and their expression. When I say the word traits, what I really mean here is your *genes*. I purposely called it traits because it's easier for you to remember four words that start with the letter T (and because thoughts, toxins, trauma, and genetics just didn't have the same ring to it). But I want to make a clear distinction here: traits come from genes on your chromosomes. Traits do not cause disease. Genes are the cause of your traits. So, if your DNA expression suddenly undergoes a biochemical change and it starts multiplying itself, well, that's cancer. The trait is the cancerous tumor, but the cause is the genes. Genetics come into play because, even when there are certain genetic issues you simply cannot overcome, you can learn ways to live better with your specific genetic makeup. Just because you have a genetic predisposition for a condition doesn't mean you have to succumb to genetic victimization. We'll cover all of this, and more, in Chapter 4.

For each T, you'll discover what can be done to mitigate symptoms, whether you're going through a major health crisis or you simply want to strengthen your body's natural immunity. Since every illness is rooted in one or more of the Four Ts, Chapter 5 takes four common illnesses and explains how each T shows up in them.

To further showcase how each T interacts with the other, Chapter 6 is dedicated to one of my patients and her journey to health via the Four Ts. You'll see how each T showed up and how we worked together to find *a better her.*

Then in Chapter 7, we'll apply the Four Ts to what happened during the 2020 COVID-19 pandemic. Viewing the pandemic while considering thoughts, toxins, trauma, and traits, I'll provide my analysis of what went incredibly wrong and what should have been avoided, especially for the next pandemic.

And finally in Chapter 8, I will offer some insight into what the future holds, the challenges I see coming, and what we can do to position ourselves and our families to resist universal composting to the best of our abilities.

More importantly, you'll find out how to implement wellness strategies to feel better, no matter where you land on the health scale. I'll show you how to stop the information overload that comes from using Dr. Google, and instead start an effective approach to health through a focused, simplified path to becoming *a better you.*

You have more power and control over your health than you realize. My goal is to present the information in a simple, clear manner to help you achieve positive change right down to the cellular level. This book is meant for educational purposes only, so it does not offer medical advice. But it will show you a different way of intimately engaging with your health, bringing to light a more focused, empowered path to move you beyond sickness into a space where true healing can begin to take place.

WHY I WROTE THIS BOOK

Since 1997, I've run a chiropractic healthcare practice in my home state of Michigan. During my tenure, I've helped patients go beyond mere symptom-based care, addressing their unique physiology in a way that allows the mind and body to find an individualized path to healing.

The process of actual, true healing is the ability for the organism (our body) to overcome its stress—to deal with it positively. Given their incredible ability to adapt and once our bodies have been given the chance, they can prosper, flourish, and grow stronger, usually without the assistance of medical intervention.

This rarely happens these days.

When someone dies, it is common for the hospice team to offer the grieving spouse something to help with the anxiety that comes with death. Most people happily take a pill of some kind, thinking it will help them, when in reality, it ends up being detrimental in the long term.

Far too often, drugs are designed to make us feel better at the sacrifice of our body. This is anti-evolutionary, it goes against nature, and it usually causes other issues. There is no such thing as side effects. I like to simply call them what they really are: effects.

For example, when we take an antibiotic shot for a bacterial infection, sure, the shot will help the infection, but the shot itself is a toxin. The body must then repair itself afterward to fix the damage done to the microbiome—the antibiotic saves life and takes life. It can take years (if ever) to improve the gut microbiome, but no one really thinks about the full spectrum of what will happen to their body when taking something as simple as an antibiotic.

I want to change that.

During my career, I unwaveringly knew that *health comes from within,* whereas our current paradigm is based on healing from the outside. In reality, health is *inside out,* and you can get to the cause of any problem by focusing on the Four Ts.

My goal is to share the knowledge I've gained over the past few decades to help you approach your health in a simple yet holistic manner, without needing a doctorate degree to understand it all. I wrote this book because I want more people to experience an "aha" moment when it comes to their health, rather than an "oh no" moment when it's too late. My hope is that this book becomes your "aha" moment, spurring you to take charge of your health via the Four Ts so you avoid hearing a doctor say, "I'm sorry to tell you that . . ."

I also want to open a new way of looking at, understanding, and talking about health among professionals and the wellness community at large. We have been approaching it all wrong, and from looking at the dismal statistics in America, something needs to change.

I'm confident that understanding the Four Ts can usher in that change.

I want to simplify the process of getting healthy, and that's what this book is about. I'm not going to use big words or confusing medical jargon. I'm going to make it so simple that, whatever you may be going through right now, and whatever challenges you've faced along your health and wellness journey, you can begin anew with a focus that's much more manageable with patient empowerment.

If that sounds good, then let's dive in, starting with a close look at the first T—our thoughts.

CHAPTER 1
THOUGHTS

WHEN HE WAS IN HIS EARLY THIRTIES, Rod told his wife exactly when he was going to die.

"I will be dead in twenty years at fifty-two, like my father," he proclaimed.

Logically, this didn't make sense. His father had died of a heart attack. That's not something you can exactly plan for.

Rod did something uncharacteristic after his father died: he spent two months privately researching sports cars—as if he had reached his midlife crisis, even though he wasn't even close, chronologically speaking. He settled on a Mercedes two-seater sports car, justifying the purchase to his wife since he believed he only had twenty more years to live.

Rod was a gifted man. He was a successful businessman who worked hard to take care of his family. He had a wonderfully supportive wife, a son, and a stepdaughter—all of whom he adored. Later, he fell naturally into his role as grandpa. His two grandchildren called him "their favorite."

Rod's brilliant mind had helped him earn a doctorate degree, but that same power of his mind was now working against him and his longevity. Because several of the males in his family had died young, he convinced himself he would encounter the same fate.

For Rod, it wasn't just a matter of belief. He *knew* he was going to die at fifty-two, and he set up his thought process to make this his reality.

There's a difference between living your life *believing*, and living your life *knowing*. Because Rod *knew* he was going to die young like his dad, he didn't feel the need to talk about it. There was no need to debate this "fact." For him, it was 100 percent concrete—this was the way it was going to be. End of story.

Being a good businessman, he retired in his forties, but he didn't treat his body well. He *knew* he would die soon, so he didn't prioritize his health and well-being.

Just shy of his fifty-second birthday, he lapsed into a diabetic coma and died.

At his service, everyone agreed on one thing: Rod had done it his way. He ended up doing exactly what he said he was going to do. He consciously created his death. He made it happen in his mind, self-fulfilling his own prophecy twenty years in the making.

Rod's story is a tragic example of what our thoughts can do to us. What if he hadn't locked in that idea? What if, a year after his father's passing, he had started to change his way of thinking, telling himself he was *not* going to die at fifty-two? Would he have taken steps to live his life differently? He was a healthcare practitioner and knew what to do.

He was also a close friend of mine, whom I miss greatly. I had planned to hand him this book, not include his story in it.

I sometimes wonder what would have happened if he had reached the age of fifty-three. Having beaten the odds he'd given himself, would he have started to take better care of himself and begun developing healthy habits? Sadly, we'll never know.

WHAT ARE THOUGHTS?

We define thoughts in many different ways, but for the purpose of addressing and identifying causes of sickness, we will view thoughts this way:

> Thoughts refer to conscious decision-making for the benefit or detriment of the human being.

The keyword here is *conscious thoughts*. I'm not referring to the subconscious, which deals with uncontrolled mind processes that lead to behaviors we don't think about. My focus in this chapter is on *conscious thoughts,* because you have the ability to change these thoughts for the benefit of your health.

The human brain is a powerful, complex organ. As we grow and develop, not only in childhood but throughout our entire lives, we actively download a wealth of information. This information comes from all around us—from the people who raise us, the culture we grow up in, the religions or philosophies we're exposed to, the schools we attend, the books we read, the personal experiences we have, and so much more. Think of it as *conscious downloading.* (Note: it's subconscious, too, but we're focusing on conscious thoughts here.)

What's more, the brain is compartmentalized. Scientists have a good grasp of where memories are stored, where speech is processed, where the brain sends signals to the foot, and so on. The basic hardware is there for most of us, and in a normal brain, this machinery helps make a thought possible.

You may be surprised to learn, however, that you do not control the exact process of making a thought. Scientists can watch a nerve cell to see what's happening *during* a thought, but they don't know how the thought first *enters* into our anatomy and physiology. At the time of this writing, it's still a mystery.

We do know, however, that the brain does not work alone. It does not operate in a vacuum. In fact, for each of us, normal brain function is completely at the mercy of our gut.

NUTRITION AND THE BRAIN

The brain is not independent from your body. In fact, the brain is at the mercy of your digestive system. There is much more to "that gut feeling" than you may think.

Your brain needs certain chemicals and substances to function its best. Where do they come from? They come from your gut. Your brain has direct communication with your digestive system through the vagus nerve. It knows what goes on down there every second of every day.

The brain interprets your health status. Reflect back to a time when you were sick or feeling unwell. How did your brain feel with a cold? Anxiety? Fever? Intestinal virus? Pain? Regardless of the specific ailment, you likely felt a bit off, mentally speaking. Mental fog is part of most diseases and infections. This is one of the reasons COVID infections cause brain fog—and also why brain fog continues to linger with long COVID. Patients with long COVID haven't fully healed from what was left by the viral damage done to the body.

While your bloodstream transports oxygen from your lungs to your brain, it also transports nutrients, phytonutrients, and hormones produced by your gut. What happens when you fill your plate with junk food with little to no nutritional value? Your brain suffers. What happens when you breathe air that's polluted? Yes, your lungs suffer, but so does your brain. To assemble your brain chemistry in a way for you to think coherently and function your best, your brain needs the right balance of nutrients and a healthy level of oxygen—with little to no toxins.

Just in case you don't know, all ultra-processed foods are toxic. Your body can't operate properly on them.

All the Ts are interdependent. For healthy thoughts that boost your well-being, it's important to protect your brain from toxins and trauma. It's also helpful to understand your genes to know how your traits may be affecting your brain and, consequently, your thought processes. Everything is interconnected. To function at its best, your brain depends on clean oxygen from your lungs and good nutrition from your gut delivered through the bloodstream—but I am getting ahead of myself. More on the other Ts coming soon.

The takeaway here is that when you treat your body well, you produce better conscious thoughts, which then lead to better choices and thus *a better you.*

THE POWER OF ADAPTATION

There is no such thing as perfection. Everyone on this planet is bound to experience challenges, hiccups, and hardship.

Not only is this okay, but this can be good for you and your health.

We need to encounter some hardship because it teaches us to adapt so we can build resilience and move forward. The body and brain need small levels of stress to adapt for the next stressor.

This is the power of adaptation.

If you are going through a challenging phase right now, take heart—we need to go through difficult times in order to overcome them. This experience then builds success that can be applied to the next problem that comes along. Life will throw you what may seem like insurmountable challenges—the loss of a job, a debilitating diagnosis, or the death of a spouse or loved one—but from what I've witnessed through my practice, those who tap into the power of adaptation learn to live with life's curveballs, even overcoming them in certain scenarios.

THE THEORY OF NEUTRALITY

On their surface, *thoughts are neutral.* We only give thoughts power when we assign feelings to them, and much of this process comes from *cultural assignment.* The specific feeling attached to a thought is what gives us the perception of good or bad, positive or negative.

But these feelings are subjective. What may be bad to you may be ineffectual to me. What you may view as negative, I may view as positive. Even if we share the same thought, our interpretation can wildly differ.

Consider how different cultures treat death. In some countries, people grieve, wear black, and struggle to adjust to their new reality without their loved ones. In other countries, people throw parades, celebrate the deceased, and show gratitude for them as they move into eternal bliss. The cultures we are raised in play a significant role in how we assign specific feelings to the thoughts that arise from our spectrum of experiences.

Thoughts are also assigned feelings depending on *point of view.* Reading a stranger's obituary may not evoke any specific feelings in you, but reading the same obituary could evoke deep sadness if you knew the person well. Conversely, if the deceased treated some family members well but was abusive to others, then the former are more likely to feel a sense of loss while the latter might feel a sense of relief. Even if we share the same thought, our own unique perspective will result in different feelings.

While thoughts on their own are neutral, we charge them with a feeling based on our beliefs. Thoughts alone don't hold power, but when the brain grabs onto the story you write and repeat for yourself, your thoughts begin to take on a life of their own—like they did for Rod when he told himself he would die at the age of fifty-two. At first, it was merely a thought, but over time, it became charged with a powerful feeling fueled by his unshakable belief, which then became his reality. He changed his brain anatomy, which led to altering his physiology.

HABITS AREN'T NEUTRAL

While thoughts are neutral until we charge them with feeling, habits are not. Every habit you develop is either beneficial or detrimental to your health and well-being. While habits form over time through consistent and repeated behaviors, they develop from feelings charged by our thoughts.

A successful health outcome requires positive cellular change. If you want to quit smoking, for example, you will have to change your mind from "I need that cigarette" to "that thing is poison." You have to transform your feelings attached to the act of smoking. Once you start doing this, your neural pattern begins to change. This change is essential to the formation of a new habit—the habit of waking up each morning and *not* automatically reaching for a cigarette, for example.

Your conscious life is driven by your thoughts. Your entire day exists as a series of positive or negative neural patterns and actions. If you're trying to lose weight, but tell yourself "I just *can't* lose weight," you risk turning this into your reality—your self-fulfilling prophecy. This thought gets charged with feeling, which then affects the action you take, which develops a specific neural pattern that strengthens over time and becomes a habit. You have to create a new neural habit to replace the old one. Our brains never entirely remove the old one either. Our brains simply create a new neural habit and may use parts of the old one. That's why recovering alcoholics often relapse after only one drink.

How can you lose weight if you tell yourself that you can't? If you're telling yourself this story repeatedly, don't be surprised to find yourself sitting down and eating half a bucket of ice cream instead of going for a walk. You're setting yourself up for failure—simply by your thoughts.

Be careful with what you tell yourself. Be mindful of your inner dialogue. Whatever you end up convincing yourself is true manifests into habits. While good habits will help develop *a better you*, bad habits will not only hold you back, but they may even shorten your lifespan.

NEUROPLASTICITY

You're probably familiar with the old adage, "you can't teach an old dog new tricks."

Well, at the time of this writing, that no longer applies. There is no age limit in our ability to improve our neuroplasticity.

Neuroplasticity is our ability to modify our neural patterns to change our actions. When it comes to improving health, neuroplasticity is our friend. The old guard initially thought our brains stopped developing at around age twenty-five and that our brains became rigid and hard to change afterward, but this has since been debunked. If you're eighty-five years old and you want to ride a bike, there's a good chance you can—as long as you're physically able, of course.

But say you're eighty-five and your legs are paralyzed—riding a bike may be out of the question. With a healthy level of neuroplasticity, though, you can achieve other goals important to you. You can be a light for other people. You can use your mind to develop a new wheelchair people can benefit from. You can become a mentor for a child. Or you can learn a new skill, like playing piano or watercolor painting.

It's about being *a better you*. When you are open to possibilities and allow yourself time to form new neural patterns, you individualize your health. This will bring a sense of optimism and confidence—because *you can* make changes, regardless of your circumstances or limitations. Whatever your condition, you still have the ability to enjoy life. You still have your gifts to share with the world.

NEURO-KNITTING HABITS

I spent countless hours watching my mother knit a specific pattern to get her desired outcome. I also watched as madness ensued when she would undo the knitting to modify the pattern. This is exactly what happens in the brain. Humans physically change their anatomy, creating new pathways to develop new habits.

Neuro-knitting is a term I use to explain what happens in the brain. If you've ever closely watched someone knit or crochet—or you're a knitter or crocheter yourself—you know what happens when a mistake is made during the process. The knitter or crocheter reverses course, takes a section of the pattern apart, and then modifies it.

This process of knitting pathways in our brains can go both ways. We can knit our way into healthy habits or unhealthy ones. Hours of repetitive drills during practice sessions make better athletes and musicians, for example. Conversely, mental addictions to food or drugs result when we develop strong physiological pathways that trigger subconscious responses, making us gravitate to actions and substances that aren't good for us.

The brain builds with repetition, so make your habits healthy ones!

And no matter where you are in life, you have what it takes to change thanks to the brain's neuroplasticity.

BONUS Ts: TIME AND STUPIDI-T

While there are Four Ts as the root to any illness or ailment, each T is also significantly affected by two other factors I call the bonus Ts: time and stupidi-T. We'll discuss how both of these impact each T.

When it comes to thoughts, time can work for you or against you. How does time affect our thoughts? Anatomically in the human mind, the more you establish and ingrain a habit or course of action, the stronger the associated neural pattern will form and the better it will run. The body adds or deletes cells to increase the speed of what it needs to get things done. Consider the habit of waking up early in the morning to work out, meditate, or journal. The more your body grows accustomed to waking up, say at 4:30 a.m., the more likely you will wake up at that hour naturally as time goes on.

The same mechanism explains why practicing sports makes us better at them. People attribute this to muscle memory, but where does that come from? It ties directly into better neural pathways created in the human brain that, over time, get stronger and faster, thus enabling people to improve at their sport. This isn't exclusive to sports, either; repetition results in physically stronger neural pathways over time in music, dance, theater, cooking, painting, learning a new language—really, just about anything humans endeavor to do.

Time is extremely important when you're trying to create a new habit. Very few people quit smoking or start a new fitness program overnight. Most people need to keep time on their side as they take steps toward a different way of living. With repeated action, new neural pathways form and strengthen. Once these pathways are in place, the new, healthier habit becomes ingrained and easier to maintain.

Our thought patterns are accompanied by biological processes. It takes time to knit firm connections between neurons in the brain and create pathways that benefit us. Remember this the next time you work on developing a healthier habit. Give yourself the gift of time.

Healing also takes time. For some of my patients, it has taken two years or longer to heal. I had a patient who suffered a stroke in the part of the brain that controlled speech. He struggled with communicating his thoughts and ideas. In order to reconnect his speech pathways, I instructed him to read limericks aloud and to write his own. With practice and commitment over several years, he slowly rebuilt those pathways and improved his speech.

For successful patients, the length of time to heal did not deter them. They were in it to win it, so they got their headspace right and took the necessary steps to improve. For some, this took months—if not years—to be *a better them*. Although some may never return to the optimum health they had before their health declined, they put in the work to maximize what their bodies were capable of in terms of healing. It takes time to get sick and time to heal.

I define stupidi-T as doing something you know is detrimental to your health and then complaining about it when your health suffers as a result.

When it comes to the stupidi-T factor, we often *knowingly* create pathways that do not benefit us, and in most cases, cause damage. That's what makes it stupid. Addiction to drugs, gambling, social media, or alcohol falls under this bonus T—but so does consuming copious amounts of unhealthy ultra-processed food. There is no difference between a heroin user and Pavlov's dogs. Whenever Pavlov rang a bell, the dogs in his experiments began to salivate subconsciously because they knew it meant feeding time. Likewise, showing a needle to an IV drug user triggers subconscious body processes that go beyond mere craving. The heroin addict believes, with every fiber of their being, they need that drug. Beyond craving, it has become a matter of life or death for them.

What screws us up is not our thoughts. Remember, a thought alone is neutral. But when we attach *excessive emotion* to a thought, we lose sight of what matters and make decisions that do not bode well. Let me explain.

The brain wants pleasure. In fact, it has an area called the satiation center. This center is responsible for your happy feelings when you're full of yummy food. After survival, pleasure is a main driver of human adaptation. Addiction is a pathway heavily tied to emotions. There is a fine line between physical and mental addiction. Given enough time and repetition, they can no longer be separated. When a person does drugs for the first time, what emotions typically surface? In most people, it is negative ones like shame or guilt. The high from the drug removes or hides those negative emotions for a while, and the user tries the drug again—mainly because they are trying to escape other negative emotions or life circumstances. When you attach negative emotion to addiction, the spiraling of the individual explodes.

Stupidi-T for thoughts is created by excessive emotion over time. What gets the human mind into trouble isn't logic, it's emotions. Emotions come in and wreck us. Like healthy habits, unhealthy ones don't develop overnight. They require time to develop too. So when we experience mental addictions, anxiety, or even fear, these conditions take root in us over time, fueled by excessive emotions attached to recurring thoughts.

We all do this, to some extent—we overthink and obsess over things we often have no control over. When this continues unchecked, we get ourselves into trouble. Many components factor in, including cultural expectations, the trauma we experienced in the past, what we eat, and more.

As you work toward improving your health and being *a better you*, keep in mind the stupidi-T factor will try to trip you up. Here's an example to clarify what I mean. Let's assume that the first time you rode a bike, you fell. Your early lessons in riding a bike left you scraped up and badly bruised. Maybe some neighborhood kids were around when you fell and they laughed at you, adding insult to injury. Now you're understandably scared of riding a bike. You've avoided it for decades. Every time you think about getting on a bicycle, your heart rate goes up, you begin perspiring, and your stomach hurts at the mere thought of it.

That's not logic—that's emotion. Logic would tell you to get on that bike and start pedaling. Emotion is what prevents you from doing so.

The majority of our issues with thought are rooted in emotion—and your body and brain don't respond the same way to logic. Emotions cause chemical reactions, and they are often supercharged by our brain and habits. Logical decisions, on the other hand, are devoid of large chemical reactions and therefore are not supercharged. Each system in your body responds to emotion, often negatively, particularly when it's an overwhelming dose. The constant emotional stress upon the body ultimately creates damage.

We are at a time and place where we like to talk about our problems, but we don't try to fix them. For healing to take place individually and collectively, this trend has to change. This is hard to do, because it requires us to become more stoic. It requires us to move away from building an identity based on victimization and instead take ownership. This allows us to move into a space where we can start to ask ourselves, "What can I do to overcome this? What can I do to thrive?"

But I believe we can do it. We need to become our own health advocates, and understanding the Four Ts is how we get there.

THE FOUR Ts MATH

To better understand the Four Ts, I've come up with an equation for each one. Now, despite these equations, there will be outliers. This demonstrates the uniqueness of the individual. But for most of us, when it comes to thoughts, the equation looks like this:

Conscious negative self-talk X repetition = amount of mental unwellness

If you have a conscious negative thought once or twice, that's fine. In fact, it's normal. You are only human after all; negative thoughts are bound to surface in your life. But if these thoughts keep coming back or increasing (meaning these negative thoughts multiply and consume most of your thinking brain), you're increasing the chances of developing some kind of mental unwellness. If you let these conscious negative thoughts continue for days, weeks, and years, you're going to manifest a disorder—whether that's anxiety, depression, paranoia, or post-traumatic stress disorder (PTSD).

Never headbutt abnormal thoughts. When they come in, let them go. Don't act on them. If you act on them, you'll create an issue. If you let your thoughts pass through you, because they are only thoughts after all, you'll exude more control over the health of your body. (This is why meditation is so beneficial: it teaches us to watch and acknowledge our thoughts, but to label them as simply thoughts and watch them pass by, like clouds on a windy day).

Respecting your thoughts (however negative) and then *replacing them* with new positive thoughts is how you level up and exude even more control over this first T. In some instances, creating positive habits that are physical in nature could be a powerful solution—lifting weights to relieve stress as opposed to drinking and smoking, for example.

The intensity of your thoughts also matters.

The strength of the negative thought X repetition = severe chronic conditions

PTSD is an example of a severe chronic condition that results from the number of times the individual thinks about the negative thought. While PTSD is usually diagnosed after a traumatic incident(s), it's the intensity of our thoughts that surface *after* the event that matters—and how long those thoughts continue before they are altered. When a veteran returns home and immediately sees a counselor to digest and process his experiences, his mind has a better chance of avoiding the creation of negative neural pathways. In contrast, if counseling doesn't start for another twenty years, then those negative neural pathways will be a lot harder to address and heal.

While PTSD is an obvious example, the strength of the negative thoughts doesn't only stem from the brutality of war, domestic violence, or other physical assault.

A negative thought can come the first time a girl looks in the mirror and thinks she's fat. Or when a group of kids calls the new foreign exchange kid stupid. If this thought is behind a powerful emotion, and the individual repeats this to themselves for months, years, or decades, then they've created some strong, negative neural pathways that will be challenging to alter.

STYLE YOUR LIFE

Your thoughts can help you improve your health and outlook, and at the same time, *you* can help your thoughts. It only takes a few seconds to start changing your thoughts for the better. Here are some practical ways to start.

Get one or more positive mentors. Everyone should have at least one mentor. In the past we referred to them as the "mothers, fathers, teachers, and preachers." Today, it can be anyone who's been there, done that—and whom you can trust. Examples may include a counselor, doctor, parent, an older sibling, or an older friend.

Seek professional counseling for complex issues. When you experience a health issue, you don't want to be left alone in the dark on the internet. You need a good support network to help you through what you need to do for your healing.

Find your people. Do you have a good support network? As social creatures, we thrive when we have solid relationships and are surrounded by a loving and supportive community.

Practice gratitude. Shifting to a mentality of gratefulness speeds up the transformation of your thought patterns to create new neural pathways. Find one to three things to be grateful for, every day, and write them down.

Practice compassion. Learn acceptance and feel forgiveness—for yourself and for others.

Be the change. There's only one person who is responsible for creating positive changes: you. Be open to personal change.

It takes time. Respect the time it takes to form new habits. You didn't get unhealthy in a day; you won't find health in one day either. Respect where you're at. It's only temporary.

Pray or meditate daily. Incorporate praying or meditating every day to ground yourself and connect with something greater than yourself.

Keep it simple and unplug. From time to time, put away the phones and electronic devices. Take off your headphones and look around. Let go of your desire for bigger payoffs and find beauty in simplicity.

Watch how you empower words. The words you use inside your head are powerful and can elicit positive or negative responses in your body. Choose your words wisely. Also, be mindful of attaching emotions to words. Words are neutral, so don't give them an identity.

Remove your temper. When we're angry, stress hormones flood our body, shutting down the rational part of your brain.

Get outside. Time spent outdoors isn't just good for the body, it's good for the mind—so get outside and enjoy fresh air, lush foliage, and sunshine on your skin.

Exercise. Exercise is medicine for the body and brain—every doctor should prescribe it! You don't need to become a gym rat—or run marathons. Find something you enjoy doing, and simply do it. Our bodies were made to move.

YOU CONTROL YOUR THOUGHTS

Our conscious thoughts are powerful, and you're the one at the wheel. You control your thoughts, and as such, you control the outcome your thoughts have on your health.

Meet Nate (not his real name). His story is quite sad, but also inspirational (if you choose). When he was in high school, he won the "Little I" award, an honor given to the graduating senior who showed the least amount of individualism and the greatest commitment to teamwork. That's the kind of person Nate was: a team player always ready to be of service.

Nate went on to become a teacher and an athletic director. One day, at the age of thirty-four, he was in the high school gym during an assembly when he passed out. The next thing he knew, he was on a plane being flown to a hospital. Nate was diagnosed with a terminal brain tumor and given a less than 5 percent chance of survival after one year. People with this type of tumor often don't make it past a year.

Without warning, his life changed in an instant. This active, energetic, and extremely fit person who worked out and looked great suddenly faced his mortality.

I don't know what thoughts went through his mind at the time of his diagnosis. What I do know is that Nate made a conscious decision to live his best life, however long that might be. Through the ensuing surgeries and procedures, he never lost his zest for life, he never wavered in his faith, and he never gave up.

True to his dedication to service and teamwork, which he had exhibited even as an eighteen-year-old winning the "Little I" award, Nate wanted the medical community to learn from his case. He wanted to help doctors find better ways to assist and support others struggling with the same disease.

What's more, he was determined to do everything in his power to live as long as possible and as best as he could. In addition to taking his medications, he also altered his diet, strictly eating foods that reduced inflammation in the body, which slowed the growth rate of cancerous cells. He did not allow anything in his body he felt was toxic.

Despite facing his mortality, Nate's diagnosis *motivated* him to take even better care of himself to prolong his life as many years as he could.

Nate did everything he could to control his thoughts. Even though he faced death, throughout all the chemo, shots, MRIs, radiation, surgeries, and more, he stayed positive. He was committed to being present for his wife and young children. He ate right, slept well, and worked doing what he loved as long as he could. He never gave up.

An avid drummer, Nate even launched a campaign to raise money so that his community had free access to a local music festival—a festival he founded. He performed at this annual festival for as long as he could. Sadly, his condition deteriorated and, although he couldn't perform live, he recorded himself playing the drums at home one last time before a brain surgery. It was the last time he played, since his abilities quickly declined afterward. Something must have told him to record that session, and he was proud of it.

Despite his disease, he lived with a positive outlook to the very end, taking his last breath at the age of forty-one, passing away peacefully in his home surrounded by family. Because of his thoughts (and then the actions that came from them), Nate not only succeeded in outliving his grim prognosis by seven years, but he also made them quality ones.

Our thoughts really have that kind of power to extend—or shorten—our lives.

Thoughts are powerful, but so is the body. The next chapter explores how the body is under attack by toxins—the second T—as well as how it works to protect us and what we can do to help our body help us.

CHAPTER 2
TOXINS

IMAGINE SITTING WITH A FRIEND at an elegant table at your favorite upscale restaurant. The two of you are enjoying an evening out, taking in the pleasant ambiance as you look through the menu. So many tantalizing dishes to choose from! Your eyes begin to scan the seafood section when your waiter returns.

"Would you like to hear about tonight's special?" he asks.

You and your friend nod.

"Our award-winning chef has prepared a special bonefish entrée cooked in a delicate cream sauce," he shares.

Both of you agree that it sounds delicious, and you decide to try it.

"Very good," your waiter responds. "We have a few options to choose from. Would you like the bonefish with antidepressants, opioid pain relievers, or blood thinners?"

"I've been feeling depressed lately," you reveal, "so I'll take the fish with the antidepressants."

"Excellent choice," your waiter responds. Turning to your friend, he asks, "And for you?"

"Strokes run in my family, so I probably should have the one with blood thinners."

What an absurd scenario, right?

Well, maybe it's not so improbable when you consider a study conducted on bonefish swimming off the coast of south Florida.[1]

---

[1] Salomé Gómez-Upegui, "Fish on Drugs: Cocktail of Medications Is 'Contaminating Ocean Food Chain,'" The Guardian (April 29, 2022), https://www.theguardian.com/environment/2022/apr/29/drugs-medications-contaminate-ocean-food-chains-fish-florida-bonefish.

Since the bonefish population had dropped by more than 50 percent since the 1980s, concerned scientists investigated to find out why. What the multiyear study revealed was shocking. The results, published in February 2022, showed alarming quantities of pharmaceuticals in the sampled bonefish.

In fact, all the bonefish tested had at least one pharmaceutical in their systems. One bonefish specimen found in the Key West region had a total of *seventeen* different pharmaceuticals in its system, some at alarmingly high concentrations.

And that's not all—researchers also discovered powerful medications within the animals bonefish typically consume, from shrimp to small fish. The study showed the very drugs we humans consume for a variety of ailments are ending up in the waters off Key West and inside the bodies of aquatic creatures living there—drugs like antidepressants, opioids, heart medicines, and antifungals, among many others. While scientists can't prove these drugs as the reason behind the bonefish population decline, the fact many different types of pharmaceuticals are present in the first place is scary—for marine life, the ecosystem, and humans alike.

Think about the people enjoying a shrimp cocktail at their favorite local tiki bars. They aren't even aware of the dangerous mix of toxins potentially present in their appetizer.

What's more alarming is that this is just one study, conducted on one species, covering one small region. The reality is everything on this planet is interconnected. Every body of water is full of pharmaceutical toxins, from the waters in Lake Michigan to the coasts of California, Australia, and South Africa. The drugs we take are contaminating the freshwater and ocean food chains, and hardly anyone seems to notice or talk about this massive problem.

WHERE ARE THESE DRUGS COMING FROM?

How are these powerful drugs that are toxic at high concentrations—or even at lower concentrations over time—ending up in lakes, rivers, and oceans?

While some invariably come from the drug manufacturing plants themselves, large quantities come from people taking these medications. In the US alone, our prescription drug usage is enormous, and it increases every year—we are talking *billions* of prescriptions with thousands of drugs to choose from.

Well, it's no wonder Key West is so polluted.

When we ingest these drugs, our bodies do not absorb them completely, meaning the body can't fully break them down and thus has to get rid of the remnants. We excrete these remnants when we go to the bathroom, and they get flushed down the toilet. Some claim the largest source of medications in water and soil comes from hospitals and clinics dumping the drugs into toilets and sinks.[2] Ultimately, these pharmaceutical substances—which wastewater plants do not have the technology to remove during the treatment process—end up in bodies of water all over the world, as well as in the soils that grow our food and the air we breathe.

And we're only talking about prescribed medications here. At the time of this writing, no major studies have been conducted on over-the-counter medications. Are medications forever chemicals?

Pharmaceuticals aren't the only toxins found in unexpected places like the waters of Key West. Many other surprising contaminants end up in our foods. For example, a 2019 study by Healthy Babies Bright Futures (HBBF) found toxic chemicals, including lead and arsenic, in 95 percent of the baby food—and they tested 168 brands![3]

Clearly, we are living in opposition to the way nature intended food to be. Making choices to help you be the best you hinges on knowing about the toxins around you and understanding what you can do to minimize their impact.

---

2   Jeff Donn, Martha Mendoza, and Justin Pritchard, "Pharmaceuticals Lurking in U.S. Drinking Water," NBC News, (March 10, 2008), https://www.nbcnews.com/health/health-news/pharmaceuticals-lurking-u-s-drinking-water-flna1c9461352.

3   "FDA Announces Action Levels for Lead in Categories of Processed Baby Foods," U.S. Food and Drug Administration (FDA), (January 24, 2023), https://www.fda.gov/news-events/press-announcements/fda-announces-action-levels-lead-categories-processed-baby-foods.

WHAT ARE TOXINS?

To better protect ourselves from toxins, we first need to understand what they are and how they affect our health. A working definition of toxins in terms of wellness is:

> Toxins are anything that, over a short or long period of time, impedes the body from functioning and being *a better you.*

There are toxins that hurt us quickly, even if we come into contact with relatively small quantities, such as carbon monoxide (which is why many homes and buildings are equipped with CO detectors) and certain venom from spider or snake bites. As humans, we've learned to recognize such toxins and protect ourselves against them.

But the toxins we're talking about in this chapter are the ones with our bonus T time component to them. When we occasionally come into contact with small quantities of toxins, our bodies usually have time to adapt. Adaptation refers to success at the cellular level. If our cells can adapt to and rise above the toxins our bodies take in, then we've achieved success in terms of health.

Think of an apple seed, which contains a substance that releases cyanide into your digestive system and blood stream. If you eat one apple, including some of the seeds, but it's the only apple you eat in a period of six months, your body has time to adapt to the toxin you've introduced into your system. You likely won't feel the effects of cyanide from the few seeds you consumed, because your body had the time to remove this toxin. But if you eat six apples a day, seeds and all, and you do this every day over several months, now you may have a problem. Cyanide builds up over time and can make you sick. High enough concentrations can even kill you.

HOW TOXINS ENTER YOUR BODY

Toxins are all around us, and they enter our bodies primarily through our mouths, noses, and skin. They can enter through a cut or a wound. They can even get in through our eyes; when we rub them, we may inadvertently push toxins, viruses, bacteria, and other foreign matter into our bodies.

During winter as a kid, did you ever break off an icicle from the roof of a home and treat it like ice cream? What a chemical treat! Those innocent looking icicles contained a lovely concoction of chemicals from the atmosphere to the oils found on the roof, and so on. Delicious!

There are several key pathways toxins take and affect you at the cellular level. These primary pathways involve:

- **Eating:** The food you ingest acquires toxins at every step of the growing and producing processes.
- **Drinking:** Generally speaking, water has been polluted by toxins from many different sources, including drugs, agricultural chemicals, microplastics, and more.
- **Breathing:** Through inhalation, you take in toxic pollutants directly from the air.
- **Absorbing:** Things that come in contact with your skin, including cosmetics, sunscreens, and cleaning supplies, contain toxins your skin absorbs into your body. This includes sun rays.

We ingest toxins when we take medicines—of course, many of these medicines (although not all) are necessary to improve the quality of our day-to-day life, minimize painful or uncomfortable symptoms, or prolong life. We may not always have the luxury of stopping these medications. But in some cases, we may have the opportunity to explore other options that could be as effective without the associated toxicity that comes from taking prescription and over-the-counter drugs. Or we may want to reduce how many pills we take while still benefiting from their medicinal value.

There are many other places where the toxins we ingest and absorb come from. Manufacturing and agriculture sectors—and even those sweet old ladies' flower gardens—are big polluters of water, contaminating nearby rivers, lakes, and other bodies of water with everything from fertilizers to toxic dyes. Many operations also release toxic particulates into the air that then fall back down and settle on the ground and in the water.

What happens when it rains? These toxic particles get washed into other areas, where they seep into the soil. You've heard of acid rain, but have you heard of acid fog or acid snow? These toxic phenomena result when acidic components, like sulfur emitted by factories, are swept by wind currents into the atmosphere where they mix with precipitation before they fall and seep into the ground.

We reside in a continual cycle of toxicity.

What happens when farmers plant seeds in tainted soil? The seedlings absorb the toxins from the soil and irrigation water. When food grows from these plants—whether melons, corn, wheat, or carrots—it also contains toxins. Even when we buy organic produce never sprayed with pesticides, the food may already contain toxins absorbed from the soil and irrigation water.

This may be why homemade baby food contains heavy metals. The organically grown peaches bought at the local farmer's market may have absorbed dangerous toxins directly from irrigation water the farmer had no idea was contaminated with those metals.

Another way we welcome toxins into our bodies is by eating ultra-processed foods. These foods are created for taste, not nutritional value—they're targeting our brains, not our bodies. Unfortunately, the majority of the adult American diet includes ultra-processed food, and our children fare worse.

While the body seeks nutrition, the brain seeks pleasure (as we mentioned in Chapter 1). Marketers and profiteers know this, and they develop food products we can't resist. The more addicted we become to our favorite junk foods and fast-food go-tos, the more money they make. Try placing a bag of chips and a plate of broccoli in front of a child—which do you think most kids will pick? You know the answer.

To reduce the quantity of toxins we ingest and increase the value of the food we eat, Americans have to change the way we view food.

Most Americans don't care about eating—they care about *being full*. Even when some well-intentioned people talk about improving school lunches for children, they don't focus on the nutritional value of the menu served. They focus on making sure kids don't feel hungry.

While, yes, addressing hunger is important, the quality of nutrition should never take second place. Getting nutritional value is far more important than feeling full. A child can feel full eating a bowl of macaroni and cheese, but that's not enough to meet the body's nutritional requirements.

In terms of nutrition, it's not a matter of one size fits all. Every person has to figure out what works for them. The diet your neighbor swears by may not work for you. The foods that work for you may or may not be the best options for your child. Everyone is unique. To start elevating your nutrition and lowering the chances of introducing toxins, we need to return to the way nature intended food to be. In my experience and from what I've seen through my practice, our bodies run well on a hunter-gatherer diet—whole foods, mostly plants, a moderate amount of protein, and zero to low sugar. The problem with the food today is that it has been chemically modified, either to enhance flavor or enhance shelf life. Our bodies have not evolved to process these chemicals. Our bodies do not recognize or know what to do with them, which is why ultra-processed food is toxic.

The bottom line: rely more on what your body *needs* than on what your pleasure-seeking brain wants.

Drinking water isn't safe either. Many people drink bottled water and believe it's a healthier option compared to tap water or other alternatives. But where did that water come from? How contaminated was the spring-fed water before it was bottled? And how hot did the water get inside the plastic bottle when it shipped from the factory to the distribution center, and then on to your neighborhood store? How hot did it get when it sat in the trunk of your vehicle all afternoon? If the water reached a certain temperature, it pulled plastic molecules out of the container, and now you're ingesting microplastics with every sip (more on this in the next section). These microplastic molecules were even found in human placentas.

Toxins can also enter through our skin. When you rub sunscreen, lotions, moisturizers, and other products directly onto your skin, or when you apply makeup on your face, the chemicals found in these products enter your bloodstream. Researchers observed that after someone applies sunscreen, chemicals can be detected in the bloodstream within a half hour—and at the time of this writing, nobody really knows what these chemicals do to the human body. If you use sunscreens, lotions, and cosmetics, apply them sparingly. Protect yourself from the sun through other means, such as by wearing hats and spending more time in the shade and less time in direct sun.

While certain products that claim to protect you from the sun are harmful, the sun itself can be a toxin too. Excessive exposure to the sun can lead to skin cancer. Sun is certainly good for us, because it gives us warmth and vitamin D, but too much of a good thing over time can become toxic.

Here's a short list of other toxins to avoid or limit exposure to:
- Radiation
- Sugar
- Alcohol
- Certain seed oils
- Certain cooking and food storage containers
- Tobacco
- Vaping
- All ultra-processed foods
- Most processed foods
- Certain types of cleaning products
- Toxic fumes (gas/oil)

A NEW TOXIN: MICROPLASTICS

We've covered toxins found in the foods we eat and the water we drink, toxins in the soil, water from production industries and agribusinesses, and toxins from pharmaceuticals, but there's a new kid on the block we are only now learning about: microplastics.

Humans have been around a long time, but microplastics are relatively new. Our bodies have not yet had the opportunity to adapt to the presence of these substances. What exactly are they?

Everywhere we look, we see things made of plastic. There are plastic bottles, bags, and buckets. Foods once stored in glass jars are now sold in plastic ones. We sit in plastic chairs, walk on carpets and wear clothes made from plastic fibers, and drink from plastic cups. We're surrounded by this material which, over time, breaks down due to heat, the sun, acidity, light, and other factors.

What scientists refer to as microplastics are the *molecules* that make up these different types of plastics we use on a daily basis. These substances break down over time and end up everywhere— in our water, our soil, and eventually our bloodstream. This is a concerning problem because we don't know what the presence of these molecules will do to us long-term. Where do they get stored? Do they remain in the bloodstream? Do they get caught in the liver? Where do all these plastic molecules go? At the time of this writing, it's a big mystery. Microplastics have even been found inside whales and at the bottom of the ocean.

Will we adapt genetically? Will other species? Only time will tell.

HOW OUR BODIES DEAL WITH TOXINS

The good news is that your body is *amazing*. It has many lines of defense, and they are found everywhere, from individual cells to organs (like the liver) to systems (like the digestive system excreting feces and urine) to something as simple as blinking our eyes. Other defenses include our skin barrier, blood-brain barrier, lymphatic system, and immune cells. The list goes on.

One such system is your microbiome. Your unique microbiome works to protect you against toxins entering into your digestive system. Your microbiome is made up of bacteria and other microorganisms that live in your digestive tract, often referred to as your gut flora. No two people on the planet have the same microbiome makeup. Each human microbiome consists of trillions of microbial cells working for you to fight off invaders, from the fungus on your cashews to the invisible mold in your coffee.

Being exposed to air, water, and food on a continual basis, your microbiome is constantly under attack. When you get food poisoning, for example, it's because you've consumed something bad for you, like a harmful strain of the *E. coli* bacteria. Your microbiome gets to work and, although unpleasant, does its job of expelling the bacteria from your body (saving your systems from further harm). Your body removes, stores, or chemically alters toxins.

But even with these systems in place, you don't want to overload them.

While your body does its best to deal with various toxins, if it gets swamped with too many, it can't adapt quickly enough, giving rise to disease and unwellness. Your body can only do so much. When you push it past its ability to protect you, you risk getting sick.

Our bodies are tough and can handle just about anything thrown at us—as long as our bodies are in an optimal state to eliminate the toxins we inhale, ingest, and absorb, and as long as we're not exposed to too much of these toxins over a long period of time.

As it stands today, however, our bodies are faced with more toxins than ever before.

BONUS Ts: TIME AND STUPIDI-T

When it comes to toxins, both of the bonus Ts—time and stupidi-T—play significant roles. Eating one cookie once a week is unlikely to hurt you, but eating an entire pack of sugary cookies every day will lead to significant health issues.

If you make poor choices and you don't give your body time to remove the toxins you've introduced, you will not be your best you.

Let's do some math!

THE FOUR Ts MATH

Just like the equation I introduced in the previous chapter on thoughts, the same equation can be applied to toxins. When it comes to the second T, the equation looks like this:

The amount of the toxin X repetition = amount of toxic load (leading to chronic or severe acute illness)

If you ingest a small amount of arsenic, for example, and this happens only once, there's not much to worry about. Your body will take care of the toxin in this small and infrequent dose. But if you happen to ingest a large dose of arsenic at once, or you ingest small amounts over a long period of time, you're looking at a trip to the emergency room—and in a worst-case scenario, death.

Now, no one voluntarily consumes arsenic, so let's apply the equation to a more common scenario. If you drink a can of sugar water or a Frappuccino every once in a while, no harm is done. Your body will adjust and deal with the glucose spike and empty calories. But if you drink one of these sugar-bombs daily for ten years, then your body won't know what to do with all the extra glucose, so it will store it as fat. As such, your insulin resistance will likely increase, and you'll develop chronic illnesses like type 2 diabetes or heart issues.

If you enjoy a glass of wine or pint of beer every once in a while on vacation or for date night with your spouse, your body can quickly and efficiently process the alcohol and you're likely to see little to no damage. But if you drink alcohol excessively over a long period of time, you open yourself up to negatively impacting your body, brain, and emotional health—from high blood pressure, heart disease, and stroke to liver disease, anxiety, and digestive problems.

Medications are also toxins, even though we often don't look at them as such. While medications help in one area, they are still foreign and toxic substances our bodies need to deal with. Abuse of these medications over time can also lead to adverse health outcomes. For example, over-the-counter nonsteroidal anti-inflammatory drugs (NSAIDs) like ibuprofen can lead to stomach ulcers if taken too often over a long period of time. But if you take the recommended dosage for a headache a handful of times a year, you don't have much to worry about.

The stupidi-T for toxins is probably the most common out of the Four Ts. We know things are bad for us, but yet we still do them. As a reminder, stupidi-T is doing something you know is detrimental to your health and then complaining about the consequences. Smokers are aware of how unhealthy their habit of smoking is, yet they continue to do it. We know excessive toxins like nicotine, sugar, and alcohol are unhealthy for us, but we continue to put them into our bodies anyway. Maybe you're lactose intolerant, but still drink milk because you like the way it tastes. Or you eat gluten even though whenever you do, your stomach and digestion screams at you later. These are all cases I would call stupid. Listen to your body. Put your body first, and respect where it is, and work with it, not against it.

STYLE YOUR LIFE

Toxins are everywhere, so it's unrealistic to think you can avoid them all. But you can be more intentional about what you put in your body and what you have in your home. Pay attention to what you're eating, drinking, inhaling, and touching, and take steps to limit your exposure to the toxins around you.

Here are just a few practical solutions you can implement to limit toxin exposure for yourself and your loved ones. Don't feel the need to do everything all at once either. Not only is that unrealistic, it can be overwhelming. Pick one thing at a time and do the best you can.

Know your water. Understand where it comes from and what is in it. Be mindful of what you use when storing it. Using a filter system can help. Avoid plastic bottles and cups.

Eat more fresh veggies. You can help your microbiome stay healthy and rid your body of toxins by consuming more fresh and lightly cooked vegetables.

Consume smaller portions. Fasting in an attempt to detoxify may not be good for you. Your body may alter its chemistry if it thinks it's going into food scarcity. Smaller portions of nutritious food throughout the day can be more beneficial.

Consistently alter your foods. Eating the same things over and over can lead to inflammation in the body that can trigger small allergic reactions. To avoid this, eat a variety of foods with different colors and textures. Consume what's seasonably available in your area.

Eat whole foods. The more that you consume foods in their pure state (not ultra-processed), the better.

Change your emotion toward food. Instead of eating to please your brain, learn to get into the pleasure of nutrition. Limit your intake of processed foods and fully avoid ultra-processed food.

Check the air quality in your home. Consider adding a few air purifiers around the house or opt for air-cleaning plants.

Think about your skin. Your skin is an organ that absorbs chemicals and toxins, so be mindful of what it touches. Research your cosmetics, lotions, shampoos, conditioners, deodorants, perfume, and sunscreen to make sure they don't contain known toxic chemicals.

DO YOUR BEST

Out of the Four Ts, most people find this one to be the most depressing or overwhelming. How are we supposed to live a toxin-free life? Answer: you can't!

But don't let that get you down. The first step is awareness. You are now aware that toxins surround us. Moving forward, *do your best* to reduce or eliminate as many as you can. Focus on the ones you have control over—cosmetics, cleaning products, replacing plastics, avoiding ultra-processed foods, and so on. And when you do absorb toxins (because we all inevitably will), have faith in your body's innate intelligence to handle them—especially if you've taken good care of your body by making healthy choices.

The majority of our mainstream diseases stem from lifestyle-oriented choices we make. Making lifestyle changes, such as opting for more natural medical treatments (where possible) and eating foods that contain more nutritional value can make a big difference in terms of being *a better you*. Reducing your exposure to toxins can help you thrive in so many areas.

Next, we'll take a look at the role the third T, trauma, plays in disease, as well as what you can do to overcome physical traumas. Being mindful of traumas you've experienced and knowing the steps you can take next can help you go from a mentality of victimization to a position of self-empowerment.

CHAPTER 3
TRAUMA

TRAUMA IS GETTING A LOT of attention as of late, and that's a good thing. People are growing more aware about psychological and emotional trauma, and then putting a plan together to address and heal from these traumas. This is admirable.

In this chapter, however, I am not referring to those traumas. When I refer to trauma, I am specifically talking about the *physical* trauma the brain and body sustain. The most common way our ancestors died was due to physical trauma—it was the number one killer. This is no longer the case, these days—thankfully.

But we still sustain various forms of trauma.

Every time you go in for a surgery, for example, your body is undergoing trauma—and it will never be the same again. In fact, most surgical procedures have steps in place to temporarily stop the body from its innate ability to save itself. The surgeon has to pause this ability in order to successfully complete the surgery.

So then the question becomes: Can the body adapt to the trauma?

Let's look at two cases that illustrate the aftermath of the trauma of surgery. In one case, a defective gallbladder was removed; in the other, a normal gallbladder was taken out. How did the patients respond?

A TALE OF TWO GALLBLADDERS

Before we get to the stories, allow me to refresh your memory about human anatomy. Sitting underneath the liver, the gallbladder is an organ that assists with the digestive process, helping your body digest fats. A normal gallbladder stores gall, also called bile, from the liver, holding on to it until it's time to inject it into the intestines for proper digestion.

When the gallbladder is missing because it has been removed, or perhaps because you were born without one, the digestive process still works, but not as well. A missing bile storage container means that fats can't be processed as effectively, so you have to be extra mindful about which foods to consume. Your body can adapt to the missing gallbladder, but it needs help. *You* must learn how to make the right dietary and lifestyle choices to prevent pain or other issues from developing.

In other words, if your gallbladder is removed, you will have abnormal digestion for the rest of your life, but because your body adapts, you just need to learn how to eat the right foods in the right quantities so you don't notice the difference.

Now on to the stories.

UNNECESSARY TRAUMA

Meet Heather, a young woman in her early twenties who sought medical help for her nausea and upset stomach. Doctors determined her gallbladder was the problem and recommended removing it. Heather never questioned the surgery and agreed to it without understanding what it would mean to her for the rest of her life.

After her procedure, she did not modify her lifestyle or her diet, and she developed cyclical vomiting syndrome, a rare disorder where she suffered repeated episodes of being sick (vomiting) and feeling sick (nausea). Her body did not adapt properly to the trauma of getting her gallbladder removed. In search of a solution to her new, postsurgical problem, she sought help and became a patient of mine.

From everything Heather shared with me, it became clear her gallbladder had not been diseased. There is a difference between how an organ looks versus how it functions. I believe her gallbladder appeared inflamed but was functioning within normal limits. After it was removed, her body did not know how to adapt properly.

Every month for a week, she would get sick, throwing up bile uncontrollably and having diarrhea. Sometimes her bouts of vomiting would last for weeks, requiring IVs for dehydration. After going through a rough week, she'd be okay for the next three weeks, and then the cycle would repeat. When she sought my help, she thought this was a normal side effect of her surgery (it isn't).

In working with Heather, I made several observations:

- The nausea and upset stomach she had prior to her surgery weren't due to a faulty gallbladder—they were the result of her eating an unhealthy, typical American diet consisting of ultra-processed foods with low nutritional value.
- She had her relatively normal functioning gallbladder removed.
- After the surgery, she saw no improvement. In fact, her digestive problems worsened and she developed cyclical vomiting syndrome.
- She did not modify her diet post-surgery.
- She was young and didn't ask questions. She failed to advocate for herself.

Sadly, Heather was even sicker after the surgery.

With some guidance, Heather slowly worked toward *a better her*. She started taking specific supplements to gently help with her stomach acidity and reduce inflammation. She also modified her diet and paid attention to how her body reacted after eating certain foods or drinks. She found even one alcoholic drink exacerbated her condition, so she quit drinking. She monitored and stayed away from allergies to specific foods. In Heather's unique case, she also had specific spinal adjustments to help restore function.

All of this should have been done *before* she opted to remove her gallbladder—but I digress.

Within a few short weeks, Heather's symptoms improved and her bouts of cyclical vomiting syndrome had diminished significantly. After a year, her body healed; no more vomiting or digestive issues. Heather now understands her dietary boundaries and is functioning at a much higher level. She can't eat cheeseburgers as much as she used to, but she has reached the point where she can get away with eating a burger occasionally without it triggering a vomiting attack.

For Heather, that's wonderful progress.

SAME BUT DIFFERENT

Ever since she was a little girl, Carol had frequent, severe stomachaches. Doctors couldn't find anything wrong, and some thought it was all in her head. One physician at a world-renowned diagnostic center even took a theatrical approach in trying to help her: as Carol sat in a clinic as a little kid, she watched him open a window and say, "I have your stomachaches here in my hand, and I'm throwing them out the window."

Unfortunately, his magic trick didn't work (I always wondered what he charged). The stomachaches continued well into adulthood. In an attempt to cope with the pain, Carol would eat her meals as fast as she could before the symptoms started. Every time she ate, she'd experience bloating, cramps, and nausea. To make matters worse, her hair was falling out too. She was miserable.

In time, a breakthrough discovery was made: Carol's gallbladder consisted of two chambers—an upper one and a lower one. This wasn't normal. A gallbladder is a unified organ. Since hers was broken up into two sections, with a significant kink in the middle, its ability to contract in response to the body's need for bile was incomplete, and this resulted in a lot of pain, bloating, and nausea.

It wasn't clear if the segmented gallbladder was deformed from birth, the result of genetics, or if it became misshapen because of some physical trauma she'd endured. Regardless of the possible cause, the result was the same—the organ wasn't working properly. Carol was already eating a healthy diet, but her gallbladder couldn't do its job properly. It had to be removed.

In Carol's case, a gallbladder removal surgery was perceived as necessary. Tests were done to determine her gallbladder was not functioning well but appeared normal—that is until the surgeon held it in his hands and said, "I've never seen a gallbladder like *this* before."

It has been more than twenty years since her gallbladder was taken out, and thanks to the surgery and her willingness to maintain a healthy diet, Carol has done very well. By avoiding greasy foods, sugars, and limiting animal proteins, Carol can today enjoy food and avoid stomachaches, experiencing reasonably good digestion even without a gallbladder. The bloating, cramps, and nausea ceased. And even her hair stopped falling out and started growing again.

This was a case of necessary trauma to the body to help Carol be *a better her*. Removing the organ was the right call. In addition, Carol understood the surgery would change her life forever—her body would have to adapt to a missing gallbladder—but it also would rid her of those awful and chronic stomach pains. By following a healthy diet afterward that supported her system, she has lived a better, healthy life.

So, in Heather's and Carol's cases, who did the healing? Who adapted to removing an organ?

WHAT IS TRAUMA?

When your body experiences physical trauma—such as surgically removing an organ, breaking a bone, or years of hard-impact exercise—your body has forever changed. It will never be the same. Physical trauma forces your body to change itself through *adaptation*, either positively or negatively.

Where possible, you want to prevent trauma. When that's not possible, as in the case with some surgeries, you want to heal trauma in the body. In cases where healing is not possible, like when removing an organ, you want to make mindful decisions to help your body adapt and thrive, despite the trauma it has experienced.

A good definition for trauma is:

Any permanent injury your body must live with and adapt to.

Examples of trauma include losing a finger or limb. Trauma can be a ligament tear, a burn wound, or a traumatic brain injury. Your body can experience trauma to tissue from a scar that's left behind years after an accident. Physical trauma can happen as a sudden, one-time occurrence, such as a ski accident that damages a knee or a farm equipment accident that results in the loss of an arm. Alternately, physical trauma can result over time. The trauma of recurring sunburns can eventually lead to the more serious trauma of skin cancer. The physical trauma caused by repetitive motions can, over time, lead to conditions such as carpal tunnel syndrome or tendonitis, for example. Illnesses can also damage our insides, leaving unseen trauma—as in the case with diseases such as polio, arthritis, and even COVID-19 (more on COVID in Chapter 7).

While any surgery will traumatize your body, sometimes surgery is the best option, as we saw in Carol's case. After doctors perform a procedure and leave you to recover, your body takes over, working to repair the damage and enabling you to heal over time.

But after surgery, your body will never be the same—it experiences a permanent change, and it does its very best to adapt. In many cases, your body can heal itself enough for you to be your best, even after going through a significant physically traumatic event.

Our bodies are amazing. They will continue to run to the best of their ability until they can't.

TRAUMA IN SCHOOL SPORTS

Increasingly, I question the benefits of youth sports. I'm all for fitness and camaraderie, but the physical trauma these teenagers go through is not worth it. The injuries I see in football players, soccer players, hockey players, boxers, and other competitive sports participants are significant—in many cases lasting a lifetime. What's the point of winning a game for an adult coach or helicopter parents if you have to suffer a lifetime of pain (or worse) as a result?

Head trauma in the form of a concussion is particularly prevalent in youth sports. Getting hit in the head can lead to not only trauma to the brain, but almost always trauma to the neck as well. The symptoms of concussion are eerily the same as the symptoms of whiplash. Far too often, the resulting trauma to the brain and neck have to be dealt with for the duration of the young person's life. Why are we putting our youth through this unnecessary, damaging physical trauma?

Concussion syndrome is a real phenomenon. Small, continual microtrauma to the tissues of the brain and body also produce a lasting effect (meaning you don't have to sustain one or two big hits, but any and all hits matter). If you played football as a young kid, and years later you experience nausea, migraines, balance issues, and other problems, there's a strong chance these symptoms that seem to come from nowhere actually come from the sports injuries you suffered to your head and neck. The neck is a source of many problems that are underdiagnosed in true concussions. I challenge you to move your head without moving your neck. Specific chiropractic care applied at the right time can alleviate many concussion symptoms and lead to proper healing.

It's time to seriously rethink competitive youth sports. Winning a game is not worth it if it leads to a destroyed body and a lifetime of health problems that could have been avoided.

BECOMING MORE MINDFUL

We can strive to be more mindful of our actions, choices, and habits to stay clear of avoidable physical trauma. For some people, eating a poor diet can lead to digestive problems and, eventually, the trauma of stomach pains and digestive system surgical procedures, as was the case with Heather. In such cases, avoiding physical trauma can be as simple as improving one's diet.

But, in some cases, trying too hard to be healthy can also lead to trauma. Overdoing it at the gym by consistently lifting heavy weights, for example, can lead to the trauma of damage to joints over time. One of the worst traumas to a body is a physical job someone works over decades to support their family. Knowledge and common sense can make a big difference in staving off injuries and surgeries.

Of course, not every instance of trauma is our fault. The body's ability to heal verges on miraculous, but our bodies do have their limits.

THE POWER OF ADAPTATION

Our bodies are incredible because they are designed to adapt—but only to a certain point. Take the example of a large laceration an employee gets at a manufacturing plant, despite taking necessary precautions. If the person is alone, lying unconscious, and their body can't stop the bleeding over time because the wound is too large, they're in trouble. They could bleed out, with the body experiencing a *limitation of matter*. It could run out of blood before it has the time to form a clot and close the wound.

The body will always strive to adapt—until the last moment possible.

When your body can no longer adapt, it essentially runs out of matter. When the white blood cells are done and stop reproducing, the body can no longer fight off infections and it can no longer self-heal. This is a limitation of matter.

There are countless examples of cases where the body can't work properly. We're supposed to have two arms and two legs to function optimally, but many people don't. They face a limitation of matter on a daily basis, and yet, they've adapted. Every day, people who are missing limbs, who have compromised cells, or who were born with DNA anomalies find ways to adapt and thrive in the face of limitations of matter. Both the body and the human spirit strive to thrive. In the realm of physical trauma, the body works to figure out what it must do to survive.

WAYS THE BODY ADAPTS

Have you noticed when astronauts return from space, they sometimes have to be transported in wheelchairs? Why is that?

In space, there is no gravity, and in the absence of this force, the body doesn't see a need for calcium for strength in the bones. It starts to pull this mineral out, slowly weakening the skeletal system. Once astronauts are back in an environment where gravity is present, the body will see a need for strengthening bones and, over time, will work to direct the calcium back.

The body will always try to adapt to its environment, conserving its resources and making the most efficient use of them. It knows much more than us.

Here's another way the body adapts to trauma. Say a person goes out into the wilderness in frigid, subfreezing weather, whether snowmobiling or cross-country skiing, and doesn't have proper protection for their hands. They will likely end up freezing their fingers, resulting in some degree of frostbite. They will lose some sensation in their fingers, and they will never be the same again. But the body can build new blood vessels around the affected areas, thus adapting and restoring some of the sensation that was lost to trauma.

Our bodies also adapt to the many stressors we encounter. In Chapter 1, I talked about how thoughts are neutral until we attach emotions to them. Similarly, stress is neutral too. The same theory of neutrality that applies to thoughts also applies to stress. It's considered favorable when it causes a positive cellular change and unfavorable when it causes a negative cellular change, such as cancer. For positive adaptation (something you want), you need positive stress. A more common form of positive stress is strength training. Physical stress under the right circumstances is good for the body. Resistance training builds muscle and strength.

But physical stress in the wrong conditions—including excessive stress and pressure—can lead to physical health problems. When you're working out or lifting weights, too much pressure on your joints can lead to physical trauma. Your knees and your shoulders shouldn't take a pounding; moderation is important. Your body needs some stress, but it also needs enough time to adapt (with rest and recovery). Exercise is excellent for the mind and body, but too much or too little can lead to problems.

Some examples of stresses that lead to positive cellular changes include saunas, red light therapy, and aerobic/anaerobic exercise. All of these activities put your body under a small amount of stress. Your body then responds by adapting to that stress so it can handle it again next time. But too much of these stressors could lead to severe health conditions.

When it comes to stress, shorter stressful events are easier to deal with than long-term stressors. While stress itself is neutral, over time, it can have a huge impact on our physical makeup. The longer your body's chromosomes, genes, proteins, and chemical processes are stressed, the worse you're going to feel.

Stressors come in countless forms, including noise pollution, an irate boss you have to deal with every day, or even something as delightful as sunshine. Twenty minutes out in the sun is fine—healthy, even. But what happens when you spend six hours in direct sunlight? Your skin is traumatized and starts to break down. If you continue to spend hours out in the sun, over time you could end up with melanoma or another type of skin cancer.

Too much radiation from the sun can cause cancer, but just enough radiation from the sun can help vitamin D work better in your body. Again, moderation is key.

It's important to balance the Four Ts to give your body what it needs to adapt and build you back, where possible, after any physical trauma. Eating nutritious foods instead of putting toxic substances into your system helps your body function its best so you can heal better. Being mentally open to your body healing itself will help you develop thought processes that support your healing. When you support your body so it can adapt following trauma, your body may even overcome genetic traits to help you be your best you.

Often, we look at people who have lost limbs and found ways to thrive as heroes, but we fail to do the same for people who overcome other types of challenges. It is remarkable to see how people adapt following traumatic experiences. It is just as remarkable to see how someone improved her physical health by changing her diet, or how somebody improved his mental health through counseling. These are important victories, too, and we need to celebrate them.

In other words, don't wait for a physical trauma to force you to adapt. Take steps now to make lifestyle choices that will help you enjoy better health. By doing so, you'll better prepare yourself in the chance you do experience emergency trauma.

YOUR BODY AT WORK

I've heard many people tell me, "I've never broken a bone in my body."

My typical reply: "Not that you're aware of."

People don't get x-rays for every slip and fall, because there's no need to. But if they did, they would likely be surprised by how many undetected fractures their bodies have endured. This is especially true with children, who are active and sustain falls from running and tripping, falling off playground equipment, stumbling downstairs, and so on. Minor breaks happen, but they heal so quickly they go unnoticed.

I was shocked to find fractures in my children's x-rays that I never knew about.

After a bone fractures, the body will immediately work to heal it on its own. This is true for both minor and major breaks. More complicated breaks, however, typically require medical attention to set properly.

Here's how the body responds to the trauma of a bone breaking. A bunch of specialized bone cells called osteoblasts arrive at the scene, filling in the gaps of the fracture and forming a large callus. The body then starts to heal that region with calcium and proteins, sealing it up. Next, cells called osteoclasts show up to fine-tune the bone, smoothing the large callus much like sandpaper smooths down a rough surface.

All this happens behind the scenes, without you even knowing. It's a pretty remarkable process of rebuilding the structural integrity that was lost due to the physical trauma of the bone fracture. Over time, the bone heals.

BONUS Ts: TIME AND STUPIDI-T

Trauma can be caused by your choices, such as pushing yourself beyond your limits when you begin to feel pain, or by taking unnecessary risks that put your body in the direct line of danger. Again, stupidi-T is doing something you know is detrimental to your health and then complaining about your health when it deteriorates.

At the same time, your ability to overcome trauma and adapt to your new reality can benefit from your choices. When you choose to eat foods that boost immunity and reduce inflammation, you help your body. When you release your addiction to cigarettes, alcohol, work, exercise, or whatever is harming you, your body gets the rest it needs, enabling it to start healing on its own.

There are some cases (but certainly not all!) where stupidi-T can be a factor in trauma. Sometimes in life, we make poor choices that result in physical trauma. Getting into a car to drive after drinking excessively can lead to an accident that results in physical injuries that could have been avoided.

It's time for some math!

THE FOUR Ts MATH

Before we get into the equation for trauma, we have to look at the two ways our body sustains trauma. The first way is through an action we repeat over time—like those runners who run for decades, leaving their joints in shambles.

The strength of the insult X prolonged time = chronic/acute condition

The same activity over a long period of time will result in trauma.

Say you get a job as a typist when you're twenty years old and you work this job for thirty years. After sitting in front of a computer typing for six hours a day for three decades, you're likely to sustain trauma, perhaps in the form of carpal tunnel in the hands, or lower back pain from sitting, or even a deteriorated disc in the neck from leaning into the screen—or all of these conditions.

Immediate traumas include surgeries, car collisions, workplace accidents, and so on. If a worker puts his hand in a combine, his arm will instantly sustain significant trauma. Climbing a mountain without a harness and then falling will cause immediate trauma (if not death).

These traumas don't occur after a long period of time, but what makes them different is the severity of the trauma. A small cut to your finger is a rather insignificant trauma that your body can deal with rather quickly. But a deeper cut could open an artery, in which case, the trauma is obviously more significant.

STYLE YOUR LIFE

Here's a list of things you can start to implement slowly to protect your body from the damaging effects of physical trauma.

Rest. Give your body the break it needs so it can heal from trauma over time without reinjuring itself.

Eat right. Your body needs nutrients so it can create the right types of matter, in optimal quantities, that it needs to repair damage.

Hydrate. We are designed from water. We need it to survive.

Mind over matter only gets you to the end of matter. A runner who runs for decades will traumatize their joints, which can lead to replacement surgery.

Use technology over physicality. Whenever possible, opt to use technology or machinery to avoid overexerting yourself and your body, which may cause trauma.

Take breaks when working. Regardless if you work a desk job or not, it's important to give your body breaks. If your job has you sitting all day, stand up every hour. Go for a short walk. If your job has you standing and on your feet all day, take breaks to get off your feet.

Work on flexibility, then strength. Include stretching in your daily routines, and lift weights a few times a week to keep your body running optimally.

Decrease sedentary lifestyle. Our bodies are meant to move. Find ways to move, even if it's minor. Park farther away from building entrances. Take the stairs instead of the elevator. Work your way up to increasing your steps. There are a multitude of ways to sprinkle activities into your daily routine without having to go to the gym or setting aside an hour or more for exercise.

Minimize repetition. Repeated movements over time can lead to chronic pain and illness, as explained in our first equation above. Keep your body guessing and do your best to avoid the same, repetitive movements—especially over long periods of time.

Minimize vibration. Excessive vibrations—from things like sound waves, loud music, equipment, etc.—damage tissues, causing minor traumas on a cellular level.

Be job safe and conscious. Accidents happen, but many of them can be avoided. If you work a job that puts you at risk for injury, take care of your Ts to arrive at work each day with a sharp and alert mind. Work to reverse or slow down any potential trauma.

Think about what you're putting your body through. Whether it's getting too much sun on vacation, not consuming enough water during the day, overtraining in the gym, or overloading on sugary treats, think about all the different ways you can improve the environment for your body to thrive.

YOU ARE MADE TO HEAL

From skin wounds to bone fractures and from chronic inflammation to severed blood vessels, your body automatically tries to heal you, restore what's bruised, broken, or infected, and rebuild itself to serve you well. Your stomach lining, for example, rebuilds itself every seven minutes. Your entire body recycles itself every seven years. For example, many people are surprised to learn that in some cases, the body can grow back new arteries and veins. If you have a clogged artery, your body may make new arteries to bypass the plugged one. Under the right circumstances, then, your body can form its own bypass!

Are you beginning to see how amazing our bodies are?

All physical trauma causes a negative cellular change in your body. So the question is: Can you still function at a near-normal level? To help your body heal, you want to do everything in your power for your body to achieve positive cellular change.

You'll need to change your lifestyle and make healthier choices to help your body adapt. You want to set up your body to thrive, even when limitations of matter exist. Just look at what many quadriplegic individuals do with their lives! Whatever trauma your body has experienced—whether you've had surgery, organ removal, broken bones and ligaments, burns, bruises, clogged arteries, or a loss of a limb—you can still support the automatic healing process within your body, so you can be your best you.

Our discussion of trauma deals with things you have some control over. It's the only T that is choice-dependent: you put yourself in the position of trauma. This differs from people who may have been born without, such as without certain limbs, organs, cell types, senses (such as hearing), or other forms of matter. This takes us to the realm of traits, which is the focus of our next chapter.

CHAPTER 4
TRAITS

WHILE THE FIRST THREE Ts—thoughts, toxins, and trauma—are significantly under your control, the fourth T is not always up to you.

Each of us is here today because our ancestors adapted genetically over time, passing these adapted genes to the next generations. Our genetics reflect our family history of adaptation across time. From our immune system to our body metabolism, we inherit a lot from our family tree. When it comes to our genes, *which give rise to our traits,* we get what we get. Does this mean that, because each of us is born with a specific set of traits, we are victims of our genes?

Absolutely not.

Even though you don't have control over which genes were passed down to you, there are many trait-related limitations you can overcome, particularly when you address the other three Ts in a positive, constructive way. Your genetic expression is not set in stone. Just as your ancestors adapted their DNA over time, you can too.

In fact, you probably already have.

ODE TO THE PRAIRIE CHICKEN

Consider the case of Joe. As a tall, lean, and fit young man, he was active and athletic. He had no major health concerns. As the years passed and he reached his thirties and forties, something changed. Genetically speaking, variants in the genes associated with his thyroid function led to him developing a thyroid condition. In other words, he was born with genes that predisposed him to developing issues with his thyroid once he reached a certain age.

He experienced a decline in his health, gaining a great deal of weight. Previously an energetic person, he became sluggish. His health declined enough to require removal of his thyroid. Without a thyroid, Joe now has to take medication to help replace some of the functionality that his thyroid previously took care of.

Joe's condition took him by surprise, and he didn't know how to deal with it. Resigning himself to his fate, he bought into what it meant to have this particular thyroid condition. In terms of the first T, his thoughts, he believed he was supposed to be sluggish and over-weight. He resigned himself to everything that came with having a slow metabolism, a lack of energy, a decreased sex drive, and a lack of motivation. He resigned himself to the supposed "fact" that, for him, losing weight was going to be difficult—maybe even impossible.

And by throwing his hands up in the air and essentially saying "I give up," Joe *became* his thyroid problem. His life turned into a living embodiment of everything he could *not* do because he no longer had a thyroid. He became the opposite of everything he once was, and not only did his health suffer, but his personal life unraveled too.

Far too many people do this. Faced with a lifelong condition developed as a result of traits that were inherited, they give up. Instead of finding a way to overcome, move forward, and be the best they can possibly be, they resign themselves to "that's just the way it is." Once they've bought into this mentality, they figure there's no need to make changes, because it's pointless.

They defeat themselves before even trying.

That's where Joe was in life. He lived life as his thyroid issue—sluggish, unable to lose weight, unmotivated—until something happened that showed him he was not as powerless as he thought.

MOTIVATED TO CHANGE

For years Joe felt defeated . . . until he met someone. A woman. Someone who had captured his attention and made him feel alive again. He wanted to get to know this person better. She was smart, witty, and beautiful—and several years younger. He reasoned that, to stand a chance with her, he needed to make some significant changes.

Suddenly motivated to slim down and boost his energy levels, Joe made changes to his diet. He started working out. Little by little, he started to see improvements. With time, his weight decreased, and he felt more energetic. With higher levels of energy, he increased his movement.

With better nutrition, physical activity, more energy, and a new outlook, Joe overcame *all Four Ts*—his self-sabotaging thoughts, the trauma of having his thyroid removed, the toxins from his diet and lifestyle, and even the traits that had given rise to his thyroid condition in the first place. Motivated by his interest in a new person, Joe found the strength and willpower to make healthy changes, which led to a better version of himself.

We can sum up his journey this way:

- Despite his overall health, he developed a thyroid condition (his body expressed traits of a disease).
- Feeling powerless, he *became* his health problem, going from being lean and active to being overweight, sluggish, and unmotivated.
- He lived this way for more than a decade, believing there was nothing he could do to improve the hand he'd been dealt.
- Then, when he met a woman who sparked his interest, he chose to implement changes to all Four Ts.
- In doing so, he overcame many of his health limitations.

Little by little, Joe got his life back. Still missing his thyroid, which he'll never get back, and still taking life-sustaining medication daily, he made lifestyle changes that led him to lose a considerable amount of weight and get fit. These changes gave him a new physique while boosting his confidence.

I love this story; he's a male prairie chicken in human form! For those of you who may not know, male prairie chickens dance for female hens each spring during courtship and mating. The better the dance moves, the more likely he will succeed in attracting a mate.

Whereas he had previously been stuck in a rut, he later felt empowered to change his life for the better. Joe left his dead-end job and found a more fulfilling one. He took back control of his health.

And the best part? His prairie chicken dance impressed his hen! He scored a date that eventually led to marriage and starting a family. The odds were against him, and for many years he believed that story. He had to contend with genetic victimization (more on this soon), the trauma of losing a vital gland, the challenge of depending on toxic but necessary medications, and his own self-defeating thoughts. But he overcame those challenges, and in the process, created a new reality beyond his wildest (prairie chicken) dreams.

WHAT ARE TRAITS?

I've been throwing the word "traits" around, and by traits I really mean genes. In this context, I define traits (genes) as:

> The accumulation of millions of years (or more) of adaptation through your ancestry to end up where you are today.

Genes form the backbone of what makes you, *you*. In the nature versus nurture dialogue, traits are pure nature. Your traits are what you are given at birth, and you'll make use of these gifts until universal composting takes them back.

With the other three Ts—thoughts, toxins, and trauma—we often see nurturing come into play. But traits are more about the biology, chemistry, and physical makeup you were born with. Some of these traits are evident as soon as you're born. Others appear over time.

You may be asking, "Well, are traits just my DNA, then?" And the answer is no. Your DNA acts as the blueprint your body follows as it grows and develops. For the most part, your DNA remains the same throughout your life; the DNA you were born with is the same DNA you die with.

As such, people often think their genetics are fixed and nothing can be done to overcome the limitations of the traits they were born with. While it is true that there are many things you cannot change, such as your eye color or blood type, you most certainly *can* change the *expression* of your genetics. Without getting too deep into the weeds, this expression is known as your RNA. While your DNA doesn't change, your RNA—the way it is *expressed*—does.

In other words, while you may not control your DNA, you may have some control over your RNA, the way your genes are *expressed*— and this is the crux of where the fourth T, traits, come into play.

To explain this further, let's visit the process of human creation. Your DNA is created and set for you the moment sperm meets egg. When you were conceived in that early stage of development, many chemical processes occurred. The chromosomes and your ancestral DNA in these processes gave rise to who you are. The body and traits you ended up with were the result of gene expression.

Not everything about you is expressed when you are born, however.

Our bodies are basically big chemistry labs. What we eat and drink, what we breathe, how much or how little we exercise, what medicines we take, how much radiation or toxins we are exposed to—everything changes our chemistry. And chemistry is what causes genetic traits to be expressed or not expressed.

Our bodies are constantly adapting genetically in ways we don't even think about. Something as simple as a callus forming is an example of how cells can change genetically to adapt. Guitar players and gymnasts, for example, develop calluses on their fingers and hands, which toughen them. This is a genetic adaptation to the conditions the cells on the hands are exposed to and the stress they're experiencing.

Another example of RNA gene expression comes via medical diagnoses. For instance, we see cellular genetic changes in people who overcome and reverse type 2 diabetes after implementing lifestyle changes (eating a healthier diet, exercising, and implementing relaxation techniques). Their DNA before they developed type 2 diabetes didn't change when they were diagnosed with the disease, nor did it change when they reversed it. What changed is the RNA—the *expression* of the disease through traits their body exhibited.

Remember, your DNA doesn't change when you are diagnosed with a disease. The disease manifests as an expression of traits, which is the RNA—and the RNA and protein synthesis can be changed.

Gene expression is a tricky thing. I recently worked with a group of young siblings with a history of childhood cancer in their family. Of these four siblings, three had cancer, one did not. Childhood cancer did not express itself in one child's genes. Why? We don't know, but we know it has to do with gene expression. Just because you have a family history of a particular disease doesn't automatically mean you'll get it. Is the likelihood higher? Maybe. Lifestyle choices play a big role in when and which genes are expressed—which explains how two siblings (even twins!) can experience different health issues in old age, depending on their lifestyle habits and how they took care of their bodies.

Gene expression comes into play as we live our lives. It can affect what we adapt to, and to what degree we can adapt. Consider two seventy-five-year-old individuals who've eaten similar diets their whole lives. One might have a great immune system and never gets sick. The other may have weak immunity and thus takes extra precautions to avoid contact with contagious people. Their different immune responses are the expression of what each has been given genetically. We saw how COVID-19 killed some people while others never even exuded a symptom. That is genetics at work (more on COVID and the Four Ts in Chapter 7).

Everybody is born with a specific gene pool, heavily influenced by our ancestors. As we age, different genes are expressed. Some people lose their hair in their twenties; others keep their hair (and even their original color) well into their seventies and beyond.

One woman in her eighties may have excellent bone density and strong bones, while another woman, also in her eighties, may have the bone density typical of someone who is a hundred, despite both of them living similar lifestyles. That's gene expression. Because of traits, some people are outliers, even if they've treated their bodies well.

You may have heard the term epigenetics, which is the study of how we change our gene expression, but not our genes. This is done through adaptation of the internal environment to meet the external environment. Get used to terms like gene editing and gene splicing—they are coming. You will be hearing a lot about them in the future. You will also be hearing about methylation—which turns chemical processes on or off in the body. Methylation of DNA molecules can change genetic expression, and we can monitor and study this through epigenetics. More and more research is being done in this field, and we have a lot to learn. Researchers have cracked the human cell and are turning toward changing DNA as the new front in the ongoing battle to treat and cure disease.

Considering our current system has roots in drilling holes in skulls to release evil spirits, I'm looking forward to what the future reveals. From miasma to bad blood to germ theory, epigenetics is the next theoretical playground. This is exciting because unlike genetic changes, epigenetic changes are reversible and do not change your DNA sequence. They can, however, change how your body expresses those sequences. What does this mean? It means we can create positive cellular changes within, which will lead to better health and *a better you*.

DON'T BE A TRAITS VICTIM

The biggest problem I see with traits and gene expression is a tendency for people to use it as an excuse. Much like Joe initially gave up on improving his health when his thyroid condition emerged, many people who are told "it's genetic" or "it runs in your family" incorrectly believe there's nothing they can do to change their lives.

They succumb to genetic victimization, which is completely unnecessary.

I'm worried these people will stop caring about their health because they've interpreted their doctor's explanation of their condition as "that's just the way it is" or "this is how I was born," and then resolve themselves to their so-called genes.

Whatever happens to run in your family, or whatever you may be diagnosed with, don't give in to genetic victimization. Look at Joe. While he succumbed to genetic victimization at first—believing there was nothing he could do to improve his condition—he later proved to himself that he had way more control over his health than he thought.

A patient of mine, a young woman, was born with a unique genetic disorder resulting in her body's inability to synthesize B vitamins. Vitamins are necessary for specific chemical reactions. Without them, your body won't function properly. As a gene-related issue, this deficiency caused several digestive issues (constipation, weight gain, etc.) and anxiety. Her body was clearly out of balance. Instead of giving into genetic victimization, she came to my practice for help. Working together, we came up with a plan to rebalance her systems. Using a specific protocol of B vitamin supplementation, over time, she built a new pathway in her body. This unique-to-her protocol allowed her to work around her genetics, and she now feels happier, more energetic, and less anxious. She didn't become her genetics; she worked around them to be *a better her.*

The way your traits are expressed is not the end all, be all! They certainly don't have to be your destiny. Don't fall prey to victimization because of the traits (genes) you've inherited. You have more power than you think.

From cystic fibrosis to Down syndrome, and from muscular dystrophy to missing limbs, many people are born with genetic conditions that can severely impact their lives, but they find ways to be their best selves. I'm sure you can think of people in your own life who fit this description.

My question, then, is this: What is your excuse? Whatever traits you were born with, there is always someone with genetics worse than you. If they can make the most of their lives, you can make the most of yours too.

SELF-CONTAINED HEALING ORGANISM

If you have beaten cancer, you've experienced a genetic change in your body. While mutations in genes under certain conditions can lead to the presence of cancer, the body is designed to get rid of cancerous cells—if you take care of your body and treat it well. Being cured of cancer involves a genetic transformation, one where the body accesses its innate ability to get rid of the old and then start again new. This process taps into and affects the genetic material within each cell.

In other words, curing cancer is a matter of *your body* getting rid of everything harmful. You may have treatments like chemotherapy and radiation to help the process, but *your body* is the one doing the work eliminating cells that have gone haywire and programming new cells to behave like they should. If it wasn't for the wonders of the human body, the chemicals used to fight cancer would never work. Your body takes charge of the healing that occurs. In fact, there is some promising research currently seeking to use the body's wisdom to fight cancer, moving away from chemotherapy and radiation.

Yes, your body is that miraculous! Give your body the credit it deserves! It is a self-contained healing organism. It needs time to adapt to trauma and stressors. It also needs rest. Rest is crucial—whether after a major injury or an intense workout. Provide your body with the time it needs to rest and heal and with the nutrition it requires to repair itself.

Having that said, the unfortunate reality is not everyone heals from cancer—the damage may be too extensive to repair, the cells may not be getting the right signal to enact genetic fixes, or inherited traits may be working against the body to block repair. But when cancer is cured, it's not the chemo that did it—it's the body that healed itself after chemically killing the cancer cells.

HOW WE NURTURE OURSELVES

Our relationship with the first three Ts has a lot to do with nurture, which has much to do with how we were raised and what we were taught.

As babies and children, the adults in our lives took care of us. They nurtured us. When we became adults, we then began to take care of and nurture ourselves. How we nurture ourselves today is significantly connected to how we respond to thoughts, toxins, and trauma.

For example, when you're eating a meal, are your thoughts telling you to hurry up and finish your food, or slow down and savor what you're eating? More often than not, these thoughts are influenced by what you learned as a kid. Slowing down is better for you. Chewing your food thoroughly helps with your digestion, in turn improving your body's nutrition and, ultimately, boosting your health. But maybe that's not how you approach mealtime.

Improving how you handle thoughts, toxins, and traumas by modifying how you care for, or nurture, yourself can help you overcome some of the limitations of your traits via positive cellular change. And when you've figured out how to make improvements in all Four Ts, you've given yourself a better chance of overcoming sickness and disease.

It comes down to getting to know and respecting who you are—because there is only one you.

BONUS Ts: TIME AND STUPIDI-T

Both time and stupidi-T play key roles in the traits arena.

Knowing you have a genetic predisposition to a disease and then continuing to abuse the previous three Ts to manifest a problem is, well, stupid. Stupidi-T can look like a person who has a high incidence of lung cancer in his family tree, or who was born with a lung issue, but chooses to smoke anyway. Smoking or vaping long enough will cause cellular changes. In short, stupidi-T is knowing certain actions are likely to negatively change your genetic expression but doing those actions anyway.

To live a healthier life and be your best you, remove any stupidi-T elements holding you back and impeding progress.

In addition, lower some of your expectations. Get out of your own way. It takes time to heal. It takes time to reverse health issues that took years (if not decades) to develop. You can change all the Ts, but only through time. Be patient.

THE FOUR Ts MATH

The equation of the fourth T includes the first three Ts:

The amount/severity of the first three Ts X time = genetic trait expression

When you focus on the first three Ts, you will see a genetic expression—but whether they are positive expressions or negative ones is based on how you feed each T. If you make healthy choices over time, you're less likely to see abnormal gene expression.

Of course, this is not a guarantee, and it comes with a bit of an asterisk. While this math checks out for the majority of us, there are certain exceptions. There are certain genetic conditions on chromosomes that are guaranteed to result in the disease. Examples include Huntington's disease, cystic fibrosis, polycystic kidney disease, and Down syndrome. But even if you are born with guaranteed genetic conditions, you still have the power within to choose how you want to live your life—so choose well!

Now that you've learned about each T, we can put it all together. The ultimate equation, which I call the *better you* restoration model, looks like this:

Improving the first three Ts over time = better trait expression = *a better you*

STYLE YOUR LIFE

Here are some practical tips to help you strengthen helpful traits and overcome potentially damaging ones.

Focus on the previous Ts. Thoughts, trauma, and toxins have a significant impact on the way your genes will be expressed. By improving the previous three Ts, your body is less likely to express negative traits.

You are not your genetics. By properly addressing thoughts, toxins, and trauma, you can change how your genes are expressed and overcome (or perhaps even avoid) some of the traits you've inherited. How you nurture yourself has a lot to do with how well you can alter your gene expression for improved health.

Don't give up. Even if your diagnosis is dire, all hope is not lost. You can take empowering steps to improve your life. You can take action to overcome the limitations of the traits you've been given. People seem to remember how we leave this planet, so make it good.

Make good decisions. Don't let stupidi-T derail you. Stop making questionable decisions. Tap into science and common sense to make smart decisions that will boost your health. In many areas, moderation is helpful.

Give yourself time. Alleviating symptoms and reversing health problems takes time. You're not going to lose a hundred pounds in ten hours. You're not going to fix any of your ailments within a week. Commit to a healthy routine and give yourself at least six months, if not a full year. At that point, reassess how you feel, and make changes to your program, as needed.

Avoid focusing on the outcome. Even if you're doing everything right with your life, you may not get the results you seek within your expected timeline. To avoid becoming a victim of time, let go of expectations and focus on the next step you have to take. Little by little, you'll get there.

LIVE YOUR BEST WITH WHAT YOU HAVE

In Chapter 1, you learned the brain seeks pleasure while the body wants nutrition. While the brain and the body can be at odds with each other at times, they want to work together so you can be your best you. Just as prairie chicken Joe conquered his thinking and got his brain and body to work together in turning his health around, even with a missing thyroid, your brain and body can learn to do what's best for *you*.

Take stock of where you are with the Four Ts. Stop blaming your traits and start working on what you can control. What improvements can you make?

When Joe took stock of his condition, he changed his thinking to "I can do better." Incrementally, he improved each T. Those improvements increased his momentum and his motivation. With commitment and time, his transformation took place. Joe's body started to express his DNA differently after he spent time addressing the other Ts and doing what was under his control. When those other Ts changed, the expression of his traits changed for the better.

In the next chapter, we'll see the Four Ts in action as we break down their roles in four of the most common illnesses in the United States.

CHAPTER 5

THE FOUR Ts IN ACTION

E VERY SICKNESS OR AILMENT can be boiled down to the Four Ts. It's rare, however, that only one T is responsible for disease. While some illnesses are rooted heavily in one T, they often overlap into one or more of the other Ts (acute conditions start with one T, whereas chronic conditions incorporate more Ts as time goes by). Some illnesses may only be rooted in three of the Four Ts. With varying degrees, each T is interconnected, and problems with one T often lead to problems in another.

But remember, this also means improving one T will lead to improvements in the others.

Now that we've covered each T on its own, it's time to see them in action. In this chapter, I'll point out how each of the Four Ts—thoughts, toxins, trauma, and traits—are rooted in four common health conditions. You will also see how our bonus Ts—time and stupidi-T—factor in.

Looking at the leading causes of death in the United States, we see heart disease, cancer, and diabetes fall among the top ten (depending on which list you use). As such, I have chosen these to highlight in this chapter. I have also included depression, because this is a common condition most of us will likely face at some point in our lives.

Let's take a look at the role thoughts, toxins, trauma, and traits play in these four common conditions, so you can better understand how each T shows up and how they are interconnected and layered.

HEART DISEASE

A thought with a strong enough emotion attached to it can indeed result in a heart attack and sudden death.

This happened in a bizarre case I read about in the later part of 2022. A woman woke up from a coma after two years and pointed to her brother as the one who had brutally attacked her. The shock, anxiety, and fear her brother felt was intense enough that, within a few days, he died from a probable heart attack. It's fascinating what excessive emotion can do to the body, isn't it?

Thankfully, this is quite rare, so let's look at a bigger example of how thoughts lead to cardiovascular issues: food.

Your thoughts are directly tied to what you choose to eat, and when we look at heart disease in America, the leading cause is poor diet. For many, heart disease develops because of a lifetime of poor eating choices. Recent studies show that 60 percent of the American diet is based on ultra-processed food lacking in nutritional value.[4] Eating poorly over an extended period of time (there's that bonus T) is a guaranteed ticket to causing problems for your heart.

Changing our thoughts about food can significantly decrease our risk of developing cardiovascular problems. This is easier said than done, mostly because the majority of folks tie emotion to their eating habits. And as we already know, emotions are tied to thoughts. If you control your thoughts, you can control your emotions, and therefore you can control what you put in your mouth.

Why is heart disease still the number one killer when we have drugs to remove cholesterol? Well, because cholesterol isn't the problem. Heart disease is not *caused* by cholesterol, but instead is simply a side effect.

Society used to think heart disease was caused by cholesterol, because we thought too much cholesterol clogged arteries, increasing the probability of heart attacks. We now know that's not true.

---

4   Anahad O'Connor, "What Are Ultra-Processed Foods? What Should I Eat Instead?" *The Washington Post*, (September 27, 2022), https://www.washingtonpost.com/wellness/2022/09/27/ultraprocessed-foods/.

The majority of heart disease is caused by decades of small inflammatory conditions, particularly inflammation of the heart and blood vessels *over time.*

Inflammatory foods run the gamut, and are specific to you and your biology, but there's one substance that is toxic for everyone: sugar. Too much sugar (and other ultra-processed foods) in the diet over time increases chronic inflammation, leading to cardiovascular issues.

Our diet is a major factor in heart disease because the standard American diet is an inflammatory nightmare. Inflammation is the number one symptom of every disease. When it comes to the American diet, our bodies do not recognize it as "food," and over time, consistent inflammation that spans decades is a recipe for cardiovascular issues.

When it comes to trauma, as far as the body is concerned, two basic types exist: immediate, which typically requires emergency care; and time-factored, which generally involves repetition. If you have a heart attack, it will cause muscle damage to your heart. Your body will have to adapt to living with less muscle related to heart function. Your body can, and in many people it does, adapt to trauma to the heart.

Ideally, though, you want to prevent a heart attack from happening in the first place. Ways to keep your heart healthy and avoid physical trauma include eating a heart-healthy diet, maintaining calm thoughts to avoid a rise in blood pressure that might trigger a heart attack (this can be achieved through meditation and breathing techniques), and avoiding direct physical hits to your chest (such as a hockey puck flung to your chest at high velocity) that could stop your heart on impact.

Heart disease is one of the conditions you may be genetically predisposed to develop, but the good news is that in many instances, the progression of heart disease can be slowed down or even prevented. In some cases, if heart disease has started, it can even be reversed.

Some people are born with heart conditions. Others are born with a liver or kidney problem and, over time, these issues can lead to heart disease. A heart condition can also develop when the body adapts poorly to the person's diet. Trauma to the heart can change your genetic expression—naturally, this is something you want to avoid.

Nutrition, fitness, and relaxation techniques help us achieve everything from lower cholesterol levels to lower blood pressure. By improving these areas, we automatically improve our heart health. With improved blood flow, the heart gets stronger and can better ward off any trait-related problems.

CANCERS

If you've been given a cancer diagnosis, how you deal with your thoughts makes a huge difference. Our thought processes can keep us alive longer, as we saw with Nate's story from Chapter 1. He lived seven years after his brain tumor diagnosis thanks in large part to his outlook and positive thought processes.

Stressed or negative thoughts will produce abnormal outcomes on the organ systems of the body. Negative thoughts over a long period of time can depress the body's immune and adrenal systems, which are needed to fight cancer.

Our bodies are efficient recyclers, constantly working on a cellular level to eliminate and recycle bad, dead, or dysfunctional cells (in a process called autophagy). This often comes as a surprise to people, but despite even the healthiest of efforts, our bodies will eventually produce cancerous cells. For those who are healthy, their body excels at actively removing and recycling these cells on a regular basis. Meanwhile, if your thought patterns are in a constant negative feedback loop—due to PTSD, high blood pressure, a terrible diet, or any number of other factors—you're overworking your adrenals. When your adrenals are under a high level of stress, the chance of those cancer cells spreading greatly increases, because your body has to work harder to recycle and eliminate abnormal cells that develop.

What isn't a surprise to most people these days is how toxins lead to cancer. Many toxins create conditions in the body that lead to the excessive growth of cancerous cells. In particular, be mindful of sugar intake, sun exposure, and excessive radiation, all of which can cause cancer.

Any chronic inflammatory condition over time can turn into cancer too. Cancer from toxicity is heavily dependent on the strength of stimulus and the amount of time. Say you eat a diet that causes inflammation in your stomach. Over time, this can lead to GERD/heartburn. Diets that consistently cause stomach inflammation and high acid can cause esophageal cells to turn cancerous.

Typically, cancers result from chemical processes that go wrong.

At the time of this writing, there is no known physical trauma that causes cancer, but I tend to disagree with this notion. Although it's harder to prove, what if the physical trauma over time changed metabolic chemistry, leading to cancer growth? I think this is plausible, and it's something for us to keep an eye on in future research.

And finally, traits are probably what most people associate with cancer. While yes, there are genetic tumors that run in families, I caution you from falling into genetic victimization. Even though your body may have genes for cancer (the DNA), that doesn't guarantee it will be expressed (the RNA). As we now know, gene expression largely depends on the other three Ts!

Certain triggers, like smoking, will negatively change a person's genetic expression over time. Generally, repetition is part of the equation. If you smoke once or twice in your life, it probably won't hurt you. But if you smoke a pack a day, every day, year after year, your altered genetics could lead to cancer, such as lung cancer or throat cancer. And if we view smoking as a physical trauma, then we answer the above question on whether physical trauma causes cancer.

While cancer can develop when cells mutate, it can also be healed when the body eliminates mutated cells, resets the cellular process, and grows new, healthy cells. Your body is an incredible machine with inner-healing intelligence, you just have to create the right conditions for it to do what it's programmed to do!

DIABETES

Type 1 diabetes is a condition people are born with or have the genetic disposition to develop, usually at a young age (traits). It is a chronic condition where the pancreas can't produce enough insulin.

Type 2 diabetes develops primarily from physical inactivity, a poor diet, or being overweight or obese. In most cases, you earn this disease. In people with this type of diabetes, the body can't break down sugars properly. The body develops insulin resistance, where the cells experience a genetic change—they become thickened to insulin as a protective measure. Insulin resistance, however, leads to a whole set of health problems.

For the purpose of this chapter, we will mainly address type 2 diabetes.

I mentioned this earlier with heart disease, but it is also true for type 2 diabetes: your thoughts are directly tied to what you choose to eat. When it comes to type 2 diabetes, we're also talking about our number one toxin: sugar.

Your blood sugar should be at a certain level for your age. In addition to contributing to previously mentioned cardiovascular issues, too much sugar over time causes blood sugar imbalances. Eating the wrong foods for a long time forces the pancreas to work too much, producing insulin and causing cellular resistance and an inability to break down sugar. Symptoms of this condition vary between individuals, but they may include being overweight, sweating profusely, smelling of sugar, lacking energy, and experiencing excessive thirst.

Changing your thinking around food and exercise can protect you against developing type 2 diabetes. Conscious eating is extremely important for reducing your risk, as well as for minimizing symptoms and regulating blood sugar if you are currently living with this condition. Conscious eating means knowing what you eat, and taking measures to improve. If you continue to eat the standard American diet, for example, and you don't care how many grams of sugar you're consuming per day, over time you will likely experience insulin resistance, which leads to type 2 diabetes. Thinking about what you eat is crucial in preventing this disease.

If you currently have this condition, changing your thought patterns can help you get your condition under control. Work with your medical or health team to change your thoughts about food and healthy living. Then turn these new thoughts into action steps to help you live a healthier life and turn your type 2 diabetes around. Going on a low-sugar diet and exercising are absolutely essential. For many, doing this can avoid a lifetime of medication, and in some cases, can even reverse this disease.

When it comes to trauma, many people with diabetes experience damage to the pancreas in the form of acute or chronic pancreatitis. Interestingly, the reverse can also happen; physical damage to the pancreas from an accident or injury can result in developing type 2 diabetes. Spinal cord trauma has also led to the onset of the disease.

In addition, people with diabetes are also at a higher risk of conditions that impair the circulatory system by degrading blood vessels. Poor blood flow can then lead to physical trauma on the legs and feet (often resulting in amputations).

If you have type 2 diabetes but you're living your best life possible, you have a good chance of reversing this disease, regardless of the genes you were born with. A better diet, a more active lifestyle, and weight loss can diminish (and even eliminate) symptoms associated with type 2 diabetes.

DEPRESSION

Most people would lump depression squarely into the first T, thoughts. But depression is an example of a disease completely dependent on all four categories.

It is not just a mental process, even though thoughts are obviously involved. Thoughts could be impacted because you're lacking neurotransmitters as a result of something vital missing from your diet. Or you may be experiencing depression because of excess toxins that entered your system years ago when you were a fetal alcohol syndrome baby.

Depression can develop from a hormonal imbalance that then affects your thought process. Some men with low levels of testosterone develop depression. Some new moms develop postpartum depression. But there are many other possible causes, too, from the foods being consumed to a genetic predisposition.

One way to protect against depression is to build inner resilience. Things will happen in life that derail us from our goals. Depression can set in when we feel we don't fit in, or when we've worked hard at something but the outcome is not what we expected. We may not have the career we hoped for, the income we wanted, or the American Dream (whatever that is these days), but it's not the end of the world. You may not get that perfect house with the white picket fence, and that's okay. Avoid attaching excessive emotions to your thought processes.

A key component of depression ties directly into what a person consumes. If you're ingesting a cocktail of toxins with your foods and beverages, your depression can worsen. By limiting the toxins you ingest, you can decrease your gut and intestinal inflammation. This will have the effect of clearing your brain and reducing symptoms of depression. Some forms of depression are chemically induced from toxins impacting the microbiome. Remember, in addition to the brain making its own chemicals, it also takes some from the digestive system via the bloodstream.

Sugars and ultra-processed foods increase inflammation; limiting intake of these foods can, over time, reduce the episodes and severity of depression. So can eating more whole foods and a well-balanced, healthy diet, which decreases inflammation. More than 80 percent of our body's serotonin is stored in enterochromaffin cells in the small intestine. Serotonin is a chemical that carries messages between nerve cells in the brain and throughout your body, and is a key player in depression. Affecting your digestion by eating toxins will severely affect these cells, which will affect your brain.

We are going to hear a lot about brain fog in the coming years. Much of it is coming from inflammation associated with our gut (digestive system) not working properly and negatively affecting the brain.

In some cases, even physical trauma to the head and neck, including concussions and whiplash, can lead to depression. Physical trauma messes with brain chemistry, which in turn can lead to mental health conditions including depression, anxiety, and obsessive-compulsive disorders.

Depression from a traumatic injury is prevalent. Imagine one minute you're walking and then the next minute you suffer a trauma that leaves you in a wheelchair.

Traits you're born with, such as genetic differences in the brain's neurotransmitters, can lead to depression. Known cellular changes in the brain lead to altered chemistry, which can then lead to depression. We are seeing these changes in the generations of some families. The only hope we have is paying attention to the first three Ts to affect the fourth one.

DON'T FORGET ABOUT STUPID

While time is a huge component for each of the above conditions, we can't forget about stupidi-T.

You can control the stupidi-T factor 100 percent of the time. The only exception here would be what children pick up and inherit from their parents. If you smoke, the chances your kids will smoke increase significantly. Same with partying, eating fast food, not exercising, and so on. Although children may make the choice to engage in these unhealthy habits, I label these instances as stupidi-T being passed down. The control factor started with the parents.

The easiest and best thing you can do for your health and longevity is to focus on your diet. I realize I keep harping on diet, but it is the most powerful aspect of health—and the one within our control. As the saying goes, you are what you eat. The body keeps track, and for it to function its best, it needs proper nutrients and minerals from real, whole foods. If you are currently suffering from any of the above conditions (or any condition, for that matter) and you don't clean up your diet, I'd call that decision stupid.

Along the same lines, if you know you are suffering from health problems, but you make no effort to change your habits or life-style to create *a better you*, then you can't complain. The fifty-year smoker can't complain about getting lung cancer. The thirty-year marathon runner can't complain of degraded joints. The twenty-year fast-food junkie can't complain of obesity and heart failure.

The majority of your health expression is because of your choices. Choose to choose well.

In the next chapter, we'll continue to explore the Four Ts in action, but this time, through a patient of mine and her journey to heal via the Four Ts.

CHAPTER 6
MEET AMELIA

Over my career, I've focused on addressing my patients' unique physiology through the Four Ts. This has allowed me to offer each patient an individualized path to healing.

Healing will look different for each of us. The process of healing is the ability of your body to overcome its challenges, setbacks, and hurdles and to deal with them as best as it can. Your body *wants* to heal, and it will go to great lengths to do so—but it can only do so much if it's not given what it needs.

Given our body's incredible ability to adapt, once we give it the chance, it can prosper, flourish, and grow stronger—usually without the assistance of medical intervention.

In this chapter, you'll meet one of my young patients, Amelia (not her real name). Through her story, I will highlight how we used the Four Ts to identify and address her unique struggles, and how we gave what her physiology needed for her to become *a better her.*

AMELIA'S JOURNEY

Amelia has dealt with debilitating stomach issues since she was in the first grade. Her symptoms worsened when she was in second grade, became particularly challenging in sixth grade, and stayed with her through her senior year of high school. Her body was perpetually in fight or flight mode.

Amelia lived in a small community and went to school with the same core group of people for years, from first grade through twelfth. A strong student who earned good grades and excelled at sports, she experienced emotional and mental stress at school due to her classmates' cliquish behavior. An independent child who did her own thing and didn't care to fit in, she became a target of their teasing and bullying, year after year.

This stress affected the first T, her thoughts (starting in her hypothalamic-pituitary-adrenal [HPA] axis). Every school day from the moment she woke up, she had to mentally prepare herself for whatever she may have encountered. "Am I going to survive this day? What do I need to say to them? How will I fight back?"

In addition to affecting her self-confidence and causing her to doubt her abilities, the thoughts brought on by other kids' bullying led directly to physiological symptoms. At school, Amelia felt angry and upset much of the time, and these turbulent thoughts manifested themselves in her body as digestive problems.

She didn't know it yet, but certain foods began acting as toxins, creating havoc within her body, and worsening her stomach pains. Amelia typically ate nutritious foods, so neither she nor her family realized her diet was interfering with her digestion.

The constant fight or flight thoughts triggered bodily reactions akin to physical trauma. Surges of hormones flooded her body, including cortisol and adrenaline, a common occurrence in people dealing with chronic stress. Excessive sports threw off her hormones too. After puberty, her periods were infrequent and irregular, another sign of physical trauma her body experienced due to hormonal imbalances caused by the stress she encountered each day. She had to wear black to hide her excessive sweating.

Finally, the trauma her body underwent led to changes in her traits. In fact, all the other Ts—thoughts, toxins, and trauma—were altering her gene expression. This process manifested itself in several physical symptoms by the time she was in college, including brittle nails, thinning hair, increased acne, and excess weight gain.

Ever since walking into her first-grade classroom and feeling the social pressure to conform, Amelia unknowingly went into battle with all Four Ts as they spiraled out of control and led to increasing health challenges.

FINDING BALANCE

My team and I started working with Amelia when she was a twenty-one-year-old college student studying health and playing college softball. She'd gone through an especially trying episode on a softball trip to another state where her stomach pain was so excruciating, she locked herself in the bathroom of the hotel room. Curled up on the floor, she called her mom and said, "I feel so sick and am in so much pain. I don't know what to do."

As we dived into Amelia's health condition, we learned she struggled with sleep. She also experienced hot flashes, anxiety, depression, and infrequent periods—all signs of postmenopause, which she was way too young for.

It was clear her body was off balance, and her body needed healing.

We began by conducting food allergy tests. We discovered she was allergic to a wide range of foods, including eggs and the protein casein, which is found in milk and other dairy products. These are both common allergens, but Amelia was also allergic to garbanzo beans, yeast, and garlic. These allergens caused inflammation in her body, which contributed to her stomach issues worsening over time.

Empowered with knowledge regarding what she could and could not eat, Amelia immediately made dietary changes, and soon her stomach pain symptoms began to subside. She also started taking gentle supplements to give her digestive system a boost while reducing inflammation in her body. She received scientific and specific chiropractic care.

Next we conducted blood tests and a hormonal panel. These revealed that Amelia's hormones were way out of balance, which explained her mood swings, missing periods, thinning hair, and postmenopausal symptoms. They also revealed adrenal fatigue. Constantly being in fight or flight mode had taken a toll on Amelia's adrenal glands. One of her symptoms associated with adrenal fatigue was physical fatigue—she felt she could never get enough sleep.

We addressed these issues with supplements to balance her hormones and boost her adrenal health. The goal of her supplementation regime was to increase her body's progesterone levels, decrease estrogen levels, and address her anemia (also caused by her hormonal imbalance).

As time went on and we saw improvements in specific areas, we rotated out supplements to continue supporting those areas while working to heal others. It was a dynamic effort on everyone's part, one that changed as weeks turned into months and months turned into years. Healing takes time and adjustment.

Two years in, Amelia achieved a significant degree of balance within her body. Her symptoms improved and many disappeared altogether.

"It took two years," she told me, "but this is the best I have felt in a long time."

Her body did all the healing. It just needed the right material and time.

A BETTER AMELIA

Slowly but surely, these efforts put Amelia back on the right path. Now twenty-three, she is no longer plagued by painful stomach pain. Her moods are better, her energy is back, and she consistently sleeps through the night and feels rested.

It took a great deal of exploration through allergen, blood, and hormonal testing to uncover what was off balance in her relatively young body. Her problem started with mental thoughts over days, weeks, and months, which affected many bodily systems. The negative effects from her thoughts were then amplified by certain foods (toxins), some of which further increased inflammation (allergens). The chronic inflammation in her body started a disease process of hormone levels in a postmenopausal state, which caused bodily trauma from chemistry changes within the body. This elaborate cycle repeated itself, causing a downstream sickness where her body expressed negative changes via her symptoms. We needed to reverse this process, which took time.

It took several different cycles of the right kinds of herbal supplements to get her body back on track. It took two years of modifications to her diet, along with a few targeted lifestyle changes. But in that time, Amelia made tremendous progress and continues to see improvement in many areas.

Treatment of her symptoms was not the answer; we needed to find the cause.

In just two years she has gone through a major transformation. Although some may think two years is a long time, considering her thoughts started as a young child, two years isn't long at all. Her journey is ongoing, but she is a much better, healthier, and happier version of herself today than she was during her elementary, middle, and high school years.

She found a *better her*.

She also feels empowered. She now knows what she is allergic to and what foods to stay away from. As her digestive system continued to heal, she reintroduced some of those items back into her diet on an occasional basis without upsetting her digestive system. Best of all, her stomach pains, brain fog, irregular periods, and angry moods are, by and large, vestiges of her past. Her hair and nails are stronger and her skin cleared up. Her weight is at a good level, too, and she can wear colors again. The anxiety attacks are gone.

Today Amelia is healthier mentally and physically, feeling greater mental clarity and higher levels of confidence. She found both journaling and yoga helpful, but most of all, she makes time for what she enjoys, giving herself plenty of time to relax, unwind, and enjoy doing her own thing.

I admire Amelia. While she learned a lot about her health and her body, she also learned how to persevere—something definitely worth developing. You'll need it when you least expect it—just as the world needed perseverance when the COVID pandemic broke out. How did the Four Ts intersect during the pandemic? That's what we'll dissect in the next chapter.

CHAPTER 7

THE FOUR Ts AND COVID-19

I F YOU THINK THAT SOUNDS like a bad name for a rock band, you're right.

In all seriousness, though, the pandemic was tough on all of us. I lost two family members to this virus, and dreadfully watched how family, friends, and patients struggled through the last several years.

When analyzing the COVID-19 response by governments across the globe using the lens of the Four Ts, it was a disaster. Governments treated the virus like a toxin that had to be eliminated at all costs, failing to consider the other Ts.

There are four major areas of influence on a human being: mental, physical, social, and spiritual. The majority of people put their time and resources into these areas. In their attempt to combat the COVID epidemic, however, most world governments focused on only one, the physical.

In both the short- and long-term view, this approach did not work well.

How we handle a global health crisis affects more than our physical health. It affects every aspect of our being—aspects that were unfortunately ignored, making things worse. And when it comes to the Four Ts, just like we do on a personal level, we can't afford to focus on just one T and ignore the rest. *They all matter.*

In this chapter, I'm going to apply the Four Ts to the pandemic, what we did wrong, what we learned, and what we should have done differently.

But first, let's briefly refresh our memory as to what happened.

COVID-19 REFRESH

If you look up the definition of COVID, you'll get something to the effect of: "a highly contagious respiratory disease caused by the SARS-CoV-2 virus."

While, yes, the virus affected a great many respiratory systems in people, the virus behind COVID-19 also had a profound effect on the heart, blood, and kidney organ systems. In most industrialized nations, cardiovascular disease is listed among the top three leading causes of death. In the United States, heart disease is the leading cause of death for men, women, and people of most racial and ethnic groups.[5] In a nation where one person dies every thirty-four seconds from cardiovascular disease, introducing COVID was not going to bode well.

And it didn't.

The COVID virus gets into our cells with the help of an enzyme found heavily in the respiratory system and kidneys. This enzyme is also high in diabetes, cardiovascular disease, and hypertension.

Once the virus is in, it instructs the invaded cell to make multiple copies of itself. This is how all viruses work. Once they've invaded, they reprogram cells, forcing them to duplicate the virus, thus creating more. Once scientists (and big pharma) learned how COVID entered the cell, they started using this method for future vaccination (and drug) trials.

The body is quite familiar with this mechanism. Your body has fought off many viral infections before. But to do so successfully, it needs to be in the best health possible. It needs a strong immune system, which you can boost (or hurt) through what you consume, what you think, and what you experience.

And this is why the virus showed up in a variety of ways. Depending on your body, your health, and the status of your Four Ts, your experience with COVID may have looked entirely different

---

5   "About Multiple Cause of Death, 1999–2020," Centers for Disease Control and Prevention, National Center for Health Statistics, CDC WONDER (accessed February 21, 2022), https://wonder.cdc.gov/mcd-icd10.html

from the experience of your spouse, your parents, your friends, or your coworkers.

While the virus affected each person differently, we then had the government handing down recommendations and mandates in an attempt to try and keep citizens safe—again, with a narrow focus on purely the physical.

Because too little was done too late—masks were not distributed immediately to everyone who needed them, information released was not transparent enough, and the most vulnerable groups were not protected properly, to name a few—we went into forced lockdowns.

This messed us up in every way—mentally, physically, socially, and spiritually.

Isolated from each other, we developed mental health issues. Education was disrupted worldwide. At the time of this writing, children are exhibiting mental health problems from not seeing their peers and not attending school in person.

Fear consumed the minds of millions. The fear surrounding what we knew and didn't know about COVID, as well as the extended isolation we endured due to lengthy lockdowns, wrecked our thoughts. Some people were too afraid to even take a healthy walk in their own neighborhoods, while others were too paralyzed by fear to walk into a grocery store to get food. Even worse, we were encouraged to report people and businesses who didn't comply with the lockdowns or mask mandates—going so far as to provide a phone number to snitch on your community.

Physically, we all suffered. Despite being on lockdown with mask mandates, people still got sick. Stuck at home, we ate too much and put on extra pounds. We ate junk food for comfort and messed up our immune systems even more. Some people drank too much alcohol. We couldn't even go to the gym to work out and exercise our bodies.

We suffered socially as well. We became paranoid of being around each other. Distrust and division grew. So did hostility toward people who weren't doing things the way we were. People wearing masks got mad at people not wearing masks. People not wearing masks got mad at people wearing masks. People became socially inept, angry, and violent toward one another.

The youngest among us, infants, also suffered socially. Masks hid adults' social expressions, and some babies couldn't learn how to read faces properly. Watching people speak is important for babies and toddlers because it teaches them about speech and how to read facial expressions. With the mask mandates, some children are now behind in their development, requiring speech therapy to catch up.[6]

We also suffered spiritually. Houses of worship closed, and even though many parishes started to worship online, church attendance decreased significantly. Churches are unlikely to ever see parishioners at pre-pandemic levels again. Our faith was tested as a nation and we failed. Our belief in the afterlife was challenged by our belief in our own mortality. We as a nation were scared.

And I'm only scratching the surface here. The many ways in which we suffered during the pandemic will affect generations to come.

WHAT WENT WRONG

Clearly, mistakes were made along the way—and I'll point some of them out—but I do not pretend to have the right answers. Believe me, I don't know what the best approach is moving forward. But I do want to share some observations in the hope that they help you make better health decisions—right now and in the future.

The first mistake was not promoting the power of our body and its incredible capabilities.

I heard a lot of talk that blamed the human body, and not enough talk about respecting it, taking care of it, and tapping into

---

6   Vanessa Clarke, Paul Lynch, and Paul Bradshaw, "Child Speech Delays Increase Following Lockdowns," BBC News (November 7, 2022), https://www.bbc.com/news/education-63373804.

its natural ability to protect us. After all, there are more viruses on Earth than there are stars in the universe. There are tons of viruses out there that we don't know about—just like COVID. A shocking study from Denmark on viruses was released in April of 2023 where they tested feces from one-year-olds. Researchers identified ten thousand viruses from this tiny subsection of humanity—many of them unknown viruses—with most of them living off bacteria to survive.[7] Despite all these viruses, we're still somehow alive. Why is that?

Because of our body's incredible ability to adapt.

Looking back through history, we see something encouraging: our bodies have never failed us as a human race. It's important to keep this in mind when confronting any pandemic or large-scale health crisis. *Our bodies are incredible*, as long as we intentionally create an environment for them to thrive.

As such, during COVID, health officials should have encouraged us to make healthy choices so our bodies could do what they're programmed to do—keep us alive. For example: they should have told us to stay active, move our bodies, and find fun ways to exercise, even when gyms were closed. Dancing, jumping jacks, or creating an obstacle course using household items to compete against family members are a few examples of getting creative.

Health officials should have told us to eat quality foods with an emphasis on dark leafy vegetables, fruits high in antioxidants, and quality protein sources full of the amino acids, vitamins, and minerals the body needs. They should have told us to drink more water and to abstain from sugary drinks and alcohol. Additionally, they should have educated us on what vitamins and supplements to take in order to help boost our body's unique protective capabilities.

Our health officials should have encouraged us to play games with family members to maintain social connection. They should

---

7   Erin Blakemore, "Scientists Identify Thousands of Unknown Viruses in Babies' Diapers," The Washington Post (April 23, 2023), https://www.washingtonpost.com/health/2023/04/23/babies-gut-diaper-study/.

have encouraged us to reach out to our friends and loved ones—not only to call (or video chat), but to also encourage them to make healthy choices. They should have told us to go outside every day for at least thirty minutes or to bask in the rays of the early morning sun to get vitamin D (no toxin-filled sunscreen necessary). And finally, they should have encouraged us to explore neutral spiritual practices—like meditation, breathwork, or even singing—to keep spirits high.

Not once during the pandemic did I hear health officials encourage any of the above.

Instead, we got fear-inducing confusion about the novel virus. One week they said masks didn't work, only to later mandate them. They confused us on how contagious the virus was, claiming it could be spread even if you didn't exude any symptoms. Every news station reported the death toll from COVID-19 on a daily basis. Some even displayed a permanent widget or ticker on their sites, keeping death front and center. Throughout the pandemic, the power of language was used to throw health-related jargon at us—words like immunization, infection, reinfection, severe infection, hospitalizations, comorbidities, intubation—all based on fear. This was a form of abuse, negatively affecting our thoughts, which then led to various poor choices.

Conversations about how the human body has what it takes to develop antibodies and fight off sickness went completely missing. In fact, the most misleading thing I heard during the pandemic was that, for the first time in the existence of humanity, we were dealing with a virus for which we had no natural immunity.

As a chiropractor and with what I understand about the human body, I knew this could not be true.

The reality is there was immunity the whole time; there just wasn't any scientific evidence to prove it. The reason our immunity wasn't discovered earlier was because scientists initially looked in the wrong place. They checked one type of cell, but eventually discovered the memory of COVID-19 stored in a different one.

And then the vaccines came out, which ended up dividing people into two groups: the vaccinated versus the unvaccinated.

As a reminder, vaccines tell your body to build immunity toward an invader. The COVID-19 vaccines gave your cells a piece of the spike protein from the virus and told them, "Remember this." Your body then built cells with a memory of the virus so it could produce antibodies.

In other words, getting vaccinated is a way to activate your body's natural immune response. When the body later sees the coronavirus again, it will know what to do: start producing antibodies to fight the invading virus.

Natural immunity—building up resistance to a virus naturally over time—does a better job of preparing the body to fight infections than vaccines do. But you risk having a more severe infection and, in some cases, dying from that infection. This is why many people chose the vaccination route. Unfortunately, we learned the hard way that it didn't matter whether you were vaccinated or not, the transmission remained the same. Regardless of your vaccination status, you were likely going to get the virus—but hopefully it wouldn't be too bad.

This knowledge was not (and still isn't) commonly known. People who got vaccinated accused those who didn't as being irresponsible. Even worse, some people accused the unvaccinated as being the reason the virus continued to spread, even though many people who got vaccinated still contracted the virus.

Regardless of your choice, it's important to note that vaccinations would not work if it weren't for your body's ability to make them work. The human body truly is magnificent—which we should have highlighted throughout the pandemic.

Another big mistake the US made was allowing one narrow branch of a much wider community to run the entire effort. The Centers for Disease Control and Prevention (CDC) set about creating strategies and advising the American public on what to do.

One of the problems with turning the task of protecting people over to one centralized organization was the narrow viewpoint that emerged. There was little room for other opinions on how to handle the pandemic. I would have liked to see specialists from several professions come together to brainstorm the best ways to move forward, think-tank style. Bringing together some of the best minds from different branches of health, medicine, psychology, chiropractic, science, virology, and clinical labs, along with hospital administrators, policy makers, and local government could have led to better, more-informed solutions best suited for each geographical region and demographic within our country.

It felt like the prevailing health model and the federal government took over the effort and mandated what we had to do—with no dissent allowed. This didn't feel scientific or prudent, especially when dealing with a virus we were still learning about. One governing body tried to control the narrative, and in doing so, began using science the wrong way—interpreting findings to fit their narrative, which is the most unscientific thing you can do. The state government in California even approved a bill to punish doctors for spreading "disinformation," even though what they said was more scientifically valid. In other words, what they said could not be unsaid, and some lost their licenses, businesses, and livelihoods.[8] As of late 2023, this bill was silently repealed.

The CDC used fear and bastardized science, which only caused more division, confusion, and death.

SWEDEN: A CASE STUDY

From the start, Sweden decided to handle the outbreak their own way (they took the Four Ts into account!), and they were attacked by the world for looking at it differently.

They kept businesses and schools open. Social distancing was advised, people were encouraged to work remotely, and people

---

8 Brendan Pierson, "California Law Aiming to Curb COVID Misinformation Blocked by Judge," Reuters (January 26, 2023), https://www.reuters.com/business/healthcare-pharmaceuticals/california-law-aiming-curb-covid-misinformation-blocked-by-judge-2023-01-26/.

with COVID symptoms were asked to self-isolate. But as a whole, the country did not shut down. Public health officials determined that, for the Swedish people, the best way to handle the virus was to develop natural immunity. It was an approach the rest of the world, for the most part, was not willing to try.

Here is an overview of what Sweden did: Early in the pandemic, social distancing was recommended, but voluntary. The country stayed open. But the vast majority of Swedes—80 percent by some estimates—did voluntarily modify their behavior to take precautions.[9] As the pandemic worsened, certain restrictions were put into place. For example, upper grade schools were closed, and visits to nursing homes were banned.

According to Worldometer (a reference website that provides counters and real-time statistics for various topics, in this case, COVID-19 cases and deaths), at the time of this writing, Sweden ranked number forty-two in terms of how many people died from COVID per population of one million. For comparison, the United States was the worst off at number one. (To clarify, ranking *lower* means more people died; ranking *higher* means fewer people died.)

Did handling the pandemic their way work out for Sweden? Yes and no.

Although Sweden did better than the United States in terms of total death toll, it still failed its elderly populations. The nation did not do enough to protect older people early in the pandemic, and as a result, the death toll for those over seventy years old was high. Tougher measures would have protected this age group and saved lives.

But Swedish children appear to have fared better than in many other countries. Primary schools stayed open, and as a result, children's mental health in Sweden is in better shape than in neighboring countries that imposed full lockdowns.

9   Emma Frans, "Did Sweden's Controversial COVID Strategy Pay Off? In Many Ways It Did – but It Let the Elderly Down," The Conversation (August 12, 2022), https:// theconversation.com/did-swedens-controversial-covid-strategy-pay-off-in-many-ways-it-did-but-it-let-the-elderly-down-188338.

Perhaps the biggest takeaway from Sweden's approach to the pandemic is that there are many ways to handle future pandemics. Before the next global health crisis hits, we have to learn from the mistakes we made during this one.

So, what did we learn?

WHAT WE LEARNED

When it came to thoughts, we learned isolation and fear dominated the general psyche, which then led to negative outcomes in all areas of what makes us human. I witnessed some people in my community become so afraid of contracting COVID-19 that they experienced what I call *a failure to thrive*—making conscious decisions that were detrimental to their health. These people didn't leave their homes, not even to get groceries. When you can't eat, move your body, or breathe fresh air, you are not going to thrive.

When it came to toxins, we learned that what you consumed made a huge difference in how your body responded to the infection. A body not overloaded with toxins and boosted by proper nutrition will fare much better when confronted with disease.

When it came to trauma, we learned that COVID-19 left some people with physical trauma and left others largely unaffected. Some individuals who lost their sense of smell or taste have not regained it, for example. And then there's long COVID, which refers to symptoms present months or years after the initial infection. In my office, I'm seeing the virus largely affecting the digestive system. Patients come in complaining of stomach pain, brain fog, a lack of energy, and a great deal of inflammation in their intestinal lining. As another long-COVID symptom, I'm also seeing women with unusually high levels of estrogen. And, of course, I'm seeing issues with the lungs, hearts, and brains with long COVID. These are all traumas the body sustained from the virus.

And when it comes to traits, we learned that they determined how our body responded to a COVID infection—or how it responded to a vaccine designed to protect us from COVID. Our traits (genes) are largely why some people got symptoms and some didn't.

Most importantly, we learned we can't focus on one T at the expense of the other three. Our efforts must boost every part of our humanity (mental, physical, social, and spiritual) while considering how to best handle all Four Ts.

WHAT WE SHOULD HAVE DONE

Looking back, it's evident the top-down approach taken with COVID-19 in the US wasn't an effective way to handle this health challenge. A better approach would have been to tackle the problem at the community level, working from the bottom up. Local committees should have been formed immediately to address the problem at a *local level*. After elected officials throughout the US got up to speed on the latest scientific discoveries about the virus, they should have dispersed that information to those local communities and let them decide the best course of action for their own residents. What were the local hospitals seeing? What did hospital administrators recommend? We should have listened to knowledgeable panels of local health authorities and empowered local leaders to act quickly.

We also should have mobilized quickly to protect the most vulnerable. Those with comorbidities were especially vulnerable to the virus—and researchers and health professionals knew that. The unhealthier you were going into the pandemic, the worse you fared. COVID exposed your body and lifestyle weaknesses through severe infection or death. As such, we should have focused our efforts on protecting older populations and protecting those with comorbidities. Too little was done in those areas. Local communities should have mobilized to protect those individuals.

And finally, we should have considered all Four Ts. We should have never lost sight of the four ways we manifest ourselves, either—mentally, physically, socially, and spiritually. These important areas that make us human were not even considered.

In a practical sense (for the next pandemic or health crisis), we need to first and foremost remind citizens of how incredible their bodies are. This is **the first T, thoughts**, in action—communities need to move out of fear paralysis and instead think of ways to provide practical help and guidance to their residents. Although most people succumb to the "fear of the unknown," we need to counter that fear with knowledge (and, in some cases, simple common sense). Instead of letting fear control us, we need to empower people with choices—choices they can make to thrive even in the scariest of circumstances.

Without fear, fellow community members would take better care of each other. We would help those who needed help. An example may look like making sure the elderly, those with a compromised immune system, and those who contracted COVID had groceries delivered to them during isolation. Delivering carefully curated, healthy groceries (even though COVID was found on groceries[10]) to the most vulnerable would have given their bodies a chance to use their natural ability to combat the illness. This would have addressed **the second T, toxins**. Instead of feeding people junk, we need to put more effort into feeding everyone food with real nutritional value to support the body.

Because we made mistakes along the way—failing to protect the most vulnerable, failing to ensure enough proper masks were available, failing to empower people to make decisions and act swiftly on the local level—we saw a great deal of **the third T, trauma**. COVID-19 has the unique ability to infiltrate every cell in the human body and cause damage. In order for masks to work properly, they needed to be worn appropriately—not to mention the proper care they necessitated in between wearing them. And as previously mentioned, the virus damaged some people's nervous system enough that their sense of taste and smell is seemingly lost forever.

On top of that, people sustained other bodily trauma from COVID-19. Patients on ventilators for days, weeks, and even

---

10 Renée Onque, "Covid-19 Can Live on These 5 Grocery Items for Days—Here's How to Consume Them Safely," CNBC (December 5, 2022), https://www.cnbc.com/2022/12/05/covid-19-can-live-on-these-5-grocery-items-for-days.html.

months sustained trauma to their mouths, throats, and noses. And who could forget the social media photos of healthcare workers who had deep marks and bruises on their faces from wearing goggles and masks as they worked unbearably long hours? Had our country been better prepared and our government made better decisions, the individual and collective trauma we experienced wouldn't have been as bad.

Our bodies are equipped to work hard to protect us. This is **the fourth T, traits**, in action. Remember your diet, habits, and mental outlook affect your traits. Even if your ancestral traits make you more susceptible to infections or experiencing more severe symptoms, you can lessen your symptoms through what you consume and how you choose to live.

Even when we don't know much about a disease and we're learning as we go, it's important to be transparent. It's necessary to own up to mistakes. It's helpful to empower people rather than scare them. In any health emergency, there is always something local communities can do to help themselves and their neighbors, but they're best off when they consider all Four Ts and come up with practical ways to boost the body's natural ability to adapt and heal.

BETTER PREPARED

We will undoubtedly face new pandemics and other health challenges in the future. It's up to us to learn from COVID-19 and get creative with solutions while moving forward with common-sense plans.

Unfortunately, we created numerous crises trying to fix the pandemic. We created political, religious, mental, physical, and social crises by bad Four Ts management. Next time, instead of these crises, I hope we have a systematic approach based on science, with voices from many different disciplines, and swift action taken at a local level to protect the most vulnerable among us. Instead of operating in crisis mode, we can operate with a real plan in place and a level head to move forward in the healthiest way possible.

And while COVID-19 was the number three killer in the United States in 2021, we can't overlook that heart disease was number one, and cancer was number two. Heart disease and cancer have been around for ages, which prompts the question: Why are we still dying from these diseases? It's clear that moving forward, we desperately need to update our approach to how we treat disease, because what we've been doing so far isn't working in making us healthier.

The future holds some serious challenges, which we will cover in the next chapter.

CHAPTER 8
WHAT THE FUTURE HOLDS

YOU'VE LIKELY HEARD THE PROVERB "It takes a village to raise a child." While this is true, a village isn't only necessary for raising children. It will also take a village to address the challenges that lie ahead.

In a thriving village, everyone has a role and works together to properly and safely produce an effective and efficient society. They cooperate with one another and work together to tackle problems that arise. Every villager takes care of what the village has for their own benefit and for the good of others.

This sounds all well and good, *but what if the village is on fire?*

This is the situation we find ourselves in now: the Four Ts are burning white-hot. We are members of a global village that is on fire in many ways, from the pollutants in our shared air, water, and soil, to the toxins we ingest through medications and over-processed foods, to negative ruminations affecting our thoughts, and the unwanted traits expressing themselves due to our current environment.

Locally, nationally, and globally, we're at risk of becoming immolated by many fires threatening our wellness. Let's take a glimpse at some of the issues we're facing today that will become even bigger challenges in the future if we do nothing about them now.

WHAT'S ON FIRE?
Toxins Are Everywhere. In Chapter 2, we looked at how toxic elements are on the rise. We consume ultra-processed foods that lack basic nutrition. We drink water that contains microplastics. We eat

seafood with high levels of pharmaceuticals. Toxins reduce the quality of the matter the body has to work with. What steps can we take, as individuals and as a whole, to make our surroundings less toxic?

Pharmaceuticals Are Out of Control. In the US, drug prescriptions increase each year, but Americans are not getting healthier. Often we are prescribed pills that may or may not work for us—nobody knows, because in many cases the research is inconclusive. The human body's ability to heal itself is much greater than any pill. How will we deal with our Big Pharma problem? Perhaps we should start by prohibiting pharmaceutical advertisements to the masses. Big Pharma names conditions using two-to-three-letter words and then markets them directly to you. The industry purposefully creates names with the letters v, x, y, and z because studies show consumers trust names with those letters. We stock up on these medications and as soon as we have a symptom, we immediately jump to our medicine cabinet. As a start, we should make it against the law for Big Pharma to advertise.

Antibiotics Resistance Is Accelerating. Overuse of antibiotics is leading to bacteria becoming more resistant and antibiotics becoming less effective. Many infections are getting harder to treat. What's our solution for when antibiotics stop working? The world is warming and new infections are coming, especially in the fungal category.

Our (Non)Healthcare System in the US Is Broken. When the number one cause pushing Americans into bankruptcy is medical bills,[11] we have a broken healthcare system. This current system is a procedures-based business that puts money first and health second. Making matters worse, the health industry employs millions of people, making change hard to usher in if it threatens the livelihoods of so many citizens. What's more, the majority of medical doctors are employees of big business—they are not to blame. What we need instead is a "Lifestyle Change" system where the

---

11 Noam N. Levey, "100 Million People in America Are Saddled with Medical Debt," *The Texas Tribune* (June 16, 2022), https://www.texastribune.org/2022/06/16/americans-medical-debt/.

emphasis is on diet and lifestyle first, pharmaceuticals second.

What are we going to do about this? Some propose Medicare for all, but is this really the answer? Is it fair for people taking good care of their bodies to pay for the medical bills of people who caused their own conditions by refusing to eat right or exercise? Whatever new system we develop, we need to make sure it's based on incentivizing good health practices and discouraging unhealthy habits. It must promote health, not perpetuate disease.

Genetic Victimization Is a Threat to Society. Relying on genetics can lead to more effective treatments for individuals. However, we can't fall into genetic victimization. When a patient hears, "You're genetically more prone to this bacterial infection because of your set of traits," there is the very real risk they will give in and give up. They may falsely believe that because they are genetically predisposed, there's nothing they can do to avoid illness and improve health. This is a dangerous attitude to adopt. We must not continue down this path.

Changing Global Weather Patterns Pose a Real Threat to Our Health. How does global warming apply to the Four Ts? It will mess up our air, land, and water, adding toxins to the resources we need for life. In turn, these changes will lead to mental stress on our populations and impair our thoughts, particularly when massive migration of populations begins to take place because of a lack of food and clean water. With excess heat, excess sun, massive flooding, and cataclysmic events, many humans will experience physical trauma. And these changes happening so quickly may impact our traits, making it challenging for humans to adapt fast enough to the environmental changes taking place around us.

Wars Harm Us. It's evident wars hurt us in countless ways. Wars degrade us in all of the Four Ts. Thoughts of foreign invaders grabbing resources bring havoc to our mental and emotional health. War leads directly to physical trauma, as seen by soldiers who return from the battlefields with missing limbs and other traumatic injuries. Some people will turn to substance abuse as a misguided way to cope, introducing toxins to the body. These toxins can in turn be passed down via fetal alcohol syndrome and babies born addicted to heroin, messing up traits for future generations. War is something we'd be wise to avoid.

Poverty Impacts Us All. When the poor can't function in society, everyone suffers. Stamping out hunger is both noble and necessary, because hungry bodies don't think well. Malnourished bodies can't fight off disease properly. Well-intentioned individuals want to make sure all our children are fed at school. This is a noble goal until you think about what schools are serving. When you look at a typical school lunch, what do you see? High concentrations of processed carbohydrates, high-fructose corn syrup, overprocessed foods like hot dogs, and greasy foods like fries. If we're going to feed our children through schools, we need to change what's on the menu, eliminating the toxins and amplifying the nutrition by adding plenty of fresh green vegetables and fruits. Otherwise, school cafeterias will give rise to more people struggling with type 2 diabetes, obesity, and heart issues.

Prisons Fail to Rehabilitate. If we want to rehabilitate prisoners and reduce crime, why not focus more on the Four Ts? If we can change the thought patterns in criminals and improve their health, it could mean safer communities with significantly less violent crime activity. Other countries are already trying this! Norway created a program to teach criminals courtesy, empathy, and social skills. Thanks to this program, they've seen a significant drop in convicted criminals reoffending.[12]

Politics Are Toxic. The political landscape has become toxic. Just listening to political coverage can be enough to raise blood pressure and create unhealthy thinking, skewing our thought processes. Can we find a way to engage with politics and bring civility into the process for a healthier outcome for everyone? Beware of catastrophic wording to create an emergency to get large bills

12 Emma Jane Kirby, "How Norway Turns Criminals into Good Neighbours," BBC News (July 7, 2019), https://www.bbc.com/news/stories-48885846.

passed that nobody has read. We also lack a moral compass, and the individual is replacing the community. We are being used for the party and not for the people.

Artificial Intelligence is Coming. With the explosion of tools like ChatGPT, artificial intelligence (AI) is guaranteed to disrupt all industries. AI is already transforming health and wellness. To give just one example, AI can analyze medical images to detect abnormalities and assist in diagnosing conditions with way better accuracy than any human. This is simply exceptional, and I see great potential in our future.

On the flip side, AI brings with it a string of challenges. It will need strict and thorough oversight, ensuring the responsible and ethical use of AI in the healthcare space and safeguarding patient interests and privacy.

To take it to a deeper level, artificial general intelligence (AGI) is also coming to a healthcare center near you. Unlike AI systems, which are designed for specific tasks, AGI steps it up as a more adaptable form of AI that can perform any task a human can do. My concern with this is that instead of depending on ourselves to improve any aspect of our lives, we will depend on AGI to do it for us.

These are all serious and complex problems—and there are many more not listed. How do we even begin to tackle these fires?

IT STARTS WITH YOU

On our own as individuals, we may feel like we can't do much—but that's not true. As simple as this may sound, putting out these various fires starts with you becoming *a better you*. A village is only as strong as its people.

So, where do *you* stand with the Four Ts?

Within your body, when one T is out of balance, the other Ts are bound to be out of balance too. They are interdependent, just as the systems in your body are interconnected. Nothing stands alone. On top of that, we also function within four primary areas of life—the mental, physical, spiritual, and social arenas.

You can't separate thoughts from toxins, because what you consume through your digestive system goes into your bloodstream and travels to your brain, affecting your thoughts. Something as simple as dehydration causes brain cells to shrink. Physical trauma from poor life decisions, previous infections, surgeries, or injuries can lead to cellular change that awakens potentially harmful traits that had been dormant within you.

Because everything that makes up you is interconnected, an imbalance in one T will create imbalance in the other Ts. But the reverse is also true: improvements in one T will lead to improvements in the other Ts over time.

Since your world is the only one you can change, you have to start there. Begin by making improvements in one T. This will have a ripple effect. Style your life! Work toward being the healthiest *you* that you can be. From there, wellness will ripple toward your family and the members of your social circles.

This is how you can prevent and stop fires from happening within your spheres of influence:

- Start with yourself. Focus on one T and begin making improvements (be sure to respect time, reduce stupidi-T, and never aim for perfection).
- Turn these improvements into habits.
- Move on to the next T and do the same.
- Repeat this for all Ts.
- Work with your loved ones and social circles to help them make improvements in the Four Ts.

Starting with the power of one, you can take concrete steps to extinguish some of the big fires our societies are dealing with today, as well as prevent new fires from starting—or at least minimize the impact of future flare-ups.

By starting with yourself and focusing on one T at a time, you can create a ripple effect of good health around the world.

CHANGE GENERATIONAL THINKING

Another powerful thing you can do to change your world and improve your health is to release yourself from the grip of generational thinking.

Without realizing it, you may have inherited an unhealthy relationship with food. For example, fifty years ago, you were considered a rock star if you provided bread and meat on the table—the symbol of success. According to society at the time, you were doing well for yourself if you provided these foods for your family. If this was how your family ate, this was normal for you and embedded into your understanding of health.

But now we're seeing cases of certain types of cancer and heart disease attributed to heavy consumption of low quality, processed meats, and type 2 diabetes; we're seeing Crohn's disease, and digestive issues attributed to heavy consumption of breads. If you consumed bread and processed meat at every meal as a child, you need to unlearn that. You must change the unhealthy grip generational thinking has on you.

A good friend of mine lost sixty pounds in six months, which also led him to wean himself off three medications. How did he do it? He shattered his generational thinking, mostly regarding what he put in his mouth. He switched from what he thought was a good diet— but which in reality was full of ultra-processed foods—and started cooking for himself using fresher, more nutritious ingredients.

When you change your world by addressing the imbalances within you, over time and across generations, you can change the whole world for the better. For you and your family, be it your biological family or your family of choice, the solutions start at home. Change yourself to change your family or immediate community, and to ultimately change the world.

HOPE FOR OUR FUTURE

It hardly even matters which T you choose to start working on. Addressing the Four Ts means addressing the root cause of your health so you can be *a better you* over the long term. Work *with* your body, not against it; it knows much more than us.

While our healthcare system is amazing at lifesaving, it is not designed to find the root causes of illness. Bypass heart surgery has saved many lives, but that surgery alone won't improve health if the patient makes no lifestyle changes moving forward. If he goes back to eating greasy burgers and fried foods, that surgery won't prolong life for very long.

Researchers continue to make progress in learning how the body works to fight disease, and also in developing ways to boost the body's natural ability to do so. For example, scientists are exploring ways to fight cancer by providing white blood cells with key pieces of information. They can now take specific white blood cells out of a person, teach these cells how to find a particular protein in the body and attack it, put these cells back into the same person, and then watch those cells destroy tumors they were taught to recognize and attack.[13] This is truly remarkable.

Breakthroughs like this mean better treatments will evolve in the near future. But this isn't the only place where I find hope. It is also found in every person who chooses to take action to improve health through lifestyle changes. Hope for the future comes from each person taking personal responsibility for our individual wholeness and focusing on making improvements in the Four Ts, one area at a time.

START A HEALTH REVOLUTION

It takes the individual to change the village. What you choose to do individually will impact not only your health, but the wholeness your family and those in your social circles experience.

The individual impacts the family. The family impacts the village. The village impacts the city. The city impacts the state. The state impacts the country. The country impacts the world.

---

13 "CAR T-Cell Therapy and Its Side Effects," American Cancer Society (March 1, 2022) https://www.cancer.org/cancer/managing-cancer/treatment-types/immunotherapy/car-t-cell1.html.

A global health revolution starts with the power of one. The following represent some simple steps you can take today to start that worldwide health revolution:

- Meditate/pray daily
- Practice a form of physical relaxation
- Exercise
- Drink clean water
- Avoid ultra-processed foods
- Improve your home's air quality
- Find a mentor or role model who practices healthy living
- Ask questions
- Research using good sources
- Think and live more positively (while respecting any negativity)

If your body mass index (BMI) is high, you can take steps today to start bringing that number down. If your blood pressure is high, you can do something right now—it could be as simple as taking five deep breaths—to create a sense of calm within your body and lower your blood pressure.[14] There is always something you can do, and it is within your reach.

Starting a health revolution that will have positive reverberations around the world is as simple as doing one thing right now to improve your health in one of the Ts. Start with your own personal health revolution and watch how your forward momentum changes the world from the bottom up.

Do it for yourself. Do it for your family. Do it for your village, state, and country.

The world is counting on you.

---

14 Hisao Mori, et al., "How Does Deep Breathing Affect Office Blood Pressure and Pulse Rate?" Hypertension Research 28 (6) (June 1, 2005): 499–504, https://doi.org/10.1291/hypres.28.499.

CONCLUSION

WHEN YOU CHANGE YOUR HEALTH, you change your life.

But you cannot change your life without changing your health.

The Four Ts have been in front of you the whole time. In the last forty years, they've appeared on most healthcare offices' patient intake forms: history of mental illness (thoughts), diet and workplace (toxins), accidents or injuries (trauma), and family history of disease or illness (traits/genes). And yet, this book is the first of its kind. Most health books pick one cause, written by experts in one area. This doesn't make them wrong; it only makes them partially right. Any future book on health (and there will be plenty) will undoubtedly deal with one (or more) of the Four Ts, and all wellness and prevention strategies will involve the Four Ts (especially the first three).

The Four Ts provide a simplified blueprint to improve your health so you can improve your life. This approach gives your body the time it needs to repair itself from whatever it has gone through. Regardless of the status of your health at this very moment, remember that your body is amazing and it contains inner healing intelligence. It wants to heal; it's up to us to set it up for success.

Overall, we need to stop putting too much emphasis on science from the outside to save the inside. We need to refocus on our body and the amazing capacity it has to heal. We boost this healing capacity when we focus on the Four Ts, give ourselves the bonus T of time, and work to eliminate stupidi-T.

In short:

- You can positively change yourself by changing your **thoughts**.
- You can positively change yourself by avoiding harmful **toxins**.
- You can positively change yourself by taking care of your body to avoid physical **trauma** (and if you have to undergo surgery, you can set your body up for success afterward).
- You can positively change yourself by working with your **traits**, as opposed to blaming them.

With the Four Ts as your roadmap, there is *always* something you can do to feel better and live healthier. You don't have to accept your current situation as your fate. Use the Four Ts as your health gurus, and they will guide you to better health.

A BETTER YOU

For too many people, healthcare has become too complicated, too overwhelming, too broken.

The system may be broken, but *you* don't have to be. You can empower yourself to better health within seconds by taking any of the Four Ts and making positive changes within that category.

It really is that simple. Start somewhere. Start today.

I wish you the best on your journey through the Four Ts. Start with one T and make changes there. Move to the next T and implement a few more healthy changes. Do this for all Four Ts, over time, and watch how you become *a better you*.

Start implementing the Four Ts with your family members and watch how those around you start to be their best too. See how this effect expands out into the world. Your actions today can even help improve traits for future generations. Nobody else can do it but you.

Share this book with others so they may benefit and join the health revolution as well. It starts with us! I also invite you to listen to my podcast, *Tapping into Uncomfortable (tappingintouncomfortable.com)*, for additional tips and more in-depth topics related to the Four Ts.

In the end, it's about being a better human. Be nice to others. Be happy with your life. Pass on good, quality daily life practices to your children, and trust that they'll pass these on to their children.

Here's to *a better you!*

ACKNOWLEDGMENTS

I WOULD LIKE TO THANK two women behind two extraordinary men. You both were instrumental in making your husbands *a better them*. I remain in awe of your strength. Thank you for letting me share your stories.

To my bride: I cannot tell you anything the poets and sages of time have not already said. What I can say, however, is that you are my lighthouse.

To my children: I have learned more from you than you have ever learned from me. You have made me better.

Dla mojej pisarki: dziękuje.

ABOUT THE AUTHOR

Reade is a living example of doing more than what he (and others) thought was possible.

He believes the only true human philosophy is hypocrisy.

He believes in positive mentors and bad examples.

He enjoys fishing.

He finds ultra-processed food frighteningly delicious.

He enjoys laughter, especially at his expense.

He believes whining should be a crime.

He respects survivors.

He likes brevity and wit. (I need to shorten this.)

He rarely reads fiction.

He whistles in the office.

He is fashion challenged.

He went from the mosh pit to the mezzanine—but he still enjoys the soothing sound of heavy metal music.

The exploding rainbow unicorn head emoji is his favorite.

He's a reformed hyperactive child and adult.

He never uses never, until he does.

He is an expected extrovert.

He is a fountain of useless knowledge, great for trivia.

He is a great example of finding yourself.

Printed in the USA
CPSIA information can be obtained
at www.ICGtesting.com
CBHW031724210524
8890CB00004B/34